INTRODUCTION

Vitamin B12, also known as cobalamin, plays a pivotal role in maintaining essential physiological functions within the human body. As one of the B vitamins, it is integral to the formation of red blood cells, the nervous system's health, and the DNA synthesis. Unlike many other vitamins, B12 is unique in its sources, primarily derived from animal products and fortified foods to a limited extent. Its deficiency can lead to a range of health complications, making it crucial for individuals to understand the significance of adequate B12 intake.

Specific populations are more susceptible to vitamin B12 deficiency. Vegetarians and vegans who abstain from or limit animal product consumption face a higher risk of insufficient B12 intake. Additionally, older adults may experience reduced stomach acid production, affecting B12 absorption. Individuals with gastrointestinal disorders, such as celiac disease or atrophic gastritis, and those who have undergone certain surgeries impacting the digestive system may also encounter challenges in absorbing B12 efficiently.

Maintaining an adequate level of vitamin B12 is

achievable through a well-balanced and diverse diet. Incorporating a variety of animal products, such as lean meats, fish, poultry, eggs, and dairy, can contribute to sufficient B12 intake. For those with dietary restrictions or absorption issues, B12 supplements are a viable option and come in various forms, including pills, sublingual tablets, and injections.

CHAPTER ONE

Understanding Vitamin B12 Deficiency

Vitamin B12 deficiency is a health condition characterized by insufficient levels of cobalamin, a water-soluble vitamin essential for various physiological functions within the human body. As a member of the B-vitamin family, B12 plays a crucial role in processes such as the formation of red blood cells, neurological function, and the synthesis of DNA.

CAUSES OF VITAMIN B12 DEFICIENCY

Vitamin B12 deficiency can arise from various factors, encompassing dietary choices, malabsorption issues, specific medical conditions, and the influence of certain medications. Understanding the multifaceted causes is essential for effective prevention and management.

A. Inadequate Dietary Intake:

• Familiar Food Sources of Vitamin B12:

• Vitamin B12 is predominantly found in animal products, including meat (beef, pork, lamb), poultry (chicken, turkey), fish (salmon, trout, tuna), dairy products (milk, cheese, yogurt), and eggs.

• Organ meats, such as liver, are wealthy sources of B12.

• Challenges for Vegetarians and Vegans:

• Individuals following plant-based diets may need help to obtain sufficient B12 due to the absence of animal products in their food choices.

• While some plant-based foods are fortified with B12, relying solely on these may pose challenges in meeting the recommended dietary intake.

B. Malabsorption Issues:

• Gastrointestinal Conditions Affecting Absorption:

• Disorders such as celiac disease, Crohn's disease, and irritable bowel syndrome (IBS) can impair the absorption of B12 by affecting the digestive system.

• Surgical procedures involving the gastrointestinal tract, including gastric bypass surgery, can also impact B12 absorption.

• Intrinsic Factor Deficiency:

• Intrinsic factor is a protein produced in the stomach that facilitates the absorption of B12 in the small intestine. A deficiency in inherent factors can impede the body's ability to absorb B12 efficiently.

C. Medical Conditions:

• Pernicious Anemia:

• Pernicious anemia is an autoimmune condition where the immune system attacks the cells in the stomach that produce intrinsic factors. As a result, inherent factor production is reduced, hindering B12 absorption.

• Atrophic Gastritis:

• Atrophic gastritis is the inflammation and thinning of the stomach lining, which can decrease intrinsic factor production and subsequently impact B12 absorption.

D. Medications Affecting B12 Absorption:

• Proton Pump Inhibitors (PPIs) and H2 Blockers: These medications, commonly used to treat conditions like acid reflux and ulcers, can reduce the production of stomach acid necessary for B12 release from food.

• Metformin: Used to manage diabetes, metformin may

interfere with B12 absorption over prolonged use.

SYMPTOMS OF VITAMIN B12 DEFICIENCY

Vitamin B12 deficiency manifests through a spectrum of symptoms that can impact various systems within the body. Recognizing these signs is crucial for early detection and appropriate intervention, preventing potential complications.

A. Fatigue and Weakness:

• One of the earliest and most common symptoms of B12 deficiency is persistent fatigue and weakness.

• Insufficient B12 hampers the production of red blood cells, leading to a decreased capacity to transport oxygen, resulting in feelings of tiredness and weakness.

B. Anemia:

• B12 deficiency often gives rise to megaloblastic anemia, a condition characterized by the production of larger-than-normal red blood cells.

• Anemic symptoms may include pale skin, shortness of breath, and a rapid heart rate as the body attempts to compensate for reduced oxygen-carrying capacity.

C. Neurological Symptoms:

• Numbness and Tingling:

• B12 is crucial for the maintenance of the nervous system, and its deficiency can result in peripheral neuropathy.

• Individuals may experience sensations of numbness and tingling, particularly in the hands and feet, as nerve function becomes compromised.

• Difficulty Walking and Balance Problems:

• B12 deficiency can impact coordination and balance, leading to difficulty walking and an increased risk of falls.

• Individuals may notice unsteadiness and a lack of coordination, which can progress if the deficiency is not addressed.

• Cognitive Disturbances:

• B12 plays a role in the synthesis of myelin, the protective covering of nerves. Deficiency may contribute to cognitive disturbances.

• Memory loss, difficulty concentrating, and mental fogginess are common cognitive symptoms associated with B12 deficiency.

Other Possible Symptoms:

• Gastrointestinal Symptoms: In some cases, individuals may experience digestive issues such as diarrhea or constipation.

• Pale or Jaundiced Skin: Anemia associated with B12 deficiency can result in a paler complexion or, in severe cases, jaundice (yellowing of the skin and eyes).

It is crucial to note that symptoms can vary in

severity and may develop gradually. Furthermore, not all individuals with B12 deficiency experience all the symptoms, making early detection challenging. Given the diverse range of manifestations, individuals exhibiting signs of fatigue, neurological symptoms, or anemia should seek medical evaluation.

GROUPS AT RISK OF VITAMIN B12 DEFICIENCY

Vitamin B12 deficiency can affect individuals across various demographics, but certain groups are particularly susceptible due to dietary preferences, physiological changes, medical conditions, or medication use. Understanding these risk factors is pivotal for targeted prevention and intervention strategies.

A. Vegetarians and Vegans:

• Rationale: Vitamin B12 is primarily found in animal products, and individuals adhering to strict vegetarian or vegan diets may have limited access to natural sources of this vitamin.

• Preventive Measures: Regular monitoring of B12 levels, consideration of fortified foods, and supplementation under healthcare guidance are essential for those adopting plant-based diets.

B. Older Adults:

• Rationale: Aging is associated with a decline in stomach acid production, which is crucial for the absorption of B12. Additionally, older people may have a reduced intake of B12-rich foods.

• Preventive Measures: Increased dietary intake of B12-rich foods, regular health check-ups, and consideration of supplementation may be recommended for older adults to address potential deficiencies.

C. Individuals with Gastrointestinal Conditions:

• Rationale: Gastrointestinal disorders such as celiac disease, Crohn's disease, or atrophic gastritis can impair the absorption of B12 in the digestive system, leading to deficiency.

• Preventive Measures: Managing underlying gastrointestinal conditions, monitoring B12 levels, and supplementation as needed are crucial for individuals with digestive disorders.

D. Patients on Certain Medications:

• Rationale:

• Proton Pump Inhibitors (PPIs) and H2 Blockers: These medications, commonly prescribed for conditions like acid reflux, reduce stomach acid production, hindering B12 absorption.

• Metformin: Used to manage diabetes, metformin may interfere with B12 absorption over prolonged use.

• Preventive Measures: Regular monitoring of B12 levels, consideration of alternative medications when possible, and B12 supplementation under medical supervision are essential for individuals on these medications.

Additional Considerations:

• Pregnant and Breastfeeding Women: Ensuring sufficient B12 intake is crucial for the health of both the mother and the developing child.

• Individuals with Pernicious Anemia: This autoimmune condition affects intrinsic factor production, necessitating B12 supplementation.

• Post-Gastric Bypass Surgery Patients: Alterations in the digestive tract may impact B12 absorption, requiring monitoring and supplementation.

DIAGNOSIS OF VITAMIN B12 DEFICIENCY

Vitamin B12 deficiency can present with a variety of symptoms, and its diagnosis involves a combination of blood tests, additional investigations to identify underlying causes, and a thorough evaluation of a patient's physical condition and medical history.

A. Blood Tests for B12 Levels:

• Serum B12 Levels: The primary diagnostic tool is measuring the concentration of vitamin B12 in the blood. A low serum B12 level is indicative of deficiency.

• Methylmalonic Acid (MMA) and Homocysteine Levels: Elevated levels of MMA and homocysteine, substances that accumulate when B12 is deficient, can provide additional confirmation of deficiency.

B. Additional Tests to Identify Underlying Causes:

• Intrinsic Factor Antibody Test: In cases where an autoimmune condition such as pernicious anemia is suspected, testing for antibodies against intrinsic factors can help confirm the diagnosis.

• Complete Blood Count (CBC): Assessing red blood cell

parameters can aid in identifying anemia and its severity.

• Gastric Analysis: For individuals with gastrointestinal conditions, gastric analysis may be performed to evaluate stomach function and intrinsic factor production.

C. Physical Examination and Medical History:

• Neurological Examination: Given the neurological implications of B12 deficiency, a thorough neurological examination may be conducted to assess symptoms such as numbness, tingling, and balance issues.

• Clinical Assessment of Anemia: Physical signs such as pale skin and nail beds, rapid heart rate, and fatigue can be indicative of anemia associated with B12 deficiency.

• Medical History: Understanding a patient's dietary habits, medical history, and any underlying conditions or medications that may impact B12 absorption is crucial for a comprehensive diagnosis.

Interpreting Results:

• Low B12 Levels: A serum B12 level below the reference range clearly indicates deficiency.

• Elevated MMA and Homocysteine Levels: Increased levels of these metabolites further support the diagnosis, especially when B12 levels are low.

• Positive Intrinsic Factor Antibody Test: The presence of antibodies against intrinsic factors suggests an autoimmune cause for B12 deficiency.

Challenges in Diagnosis:

• Subclinical Deficiency: Some individuals may have B12 levels within the reference range but still experience symptoms. Clinical judgment, symptoms, and additional tests may be considered for diagnosis in such cases.

• False Normal Levels: Conditions like folate deficiency can mask the actual severity of B12 deficiency, emphasizing the need for a comprehensive assessment.

TREATMENT AND MANAGEMENT OF VITAMIN B12 DEFICIENCY

Effectively addressing vitamin B12 deficiency involves a combination of dietary changes, supplementation, and targeted interventions to manage underlying causes. This multifaceted approach aims to restore optimal B12 levels, alleviate symptoms, and prevent complications.

A. Dietary Changes:

• Foods Rich in Vitamin B12:

• Include B12-rich foods in the diet, emphasizing animal products such as meat (beef, pork, lamb), poultry (chicken, turkey), fish (salmon, trout, tuna), dairy products (milk, cheese, yogurt), and eggs.

• Organ meats, like liver, are particularly dense sources of B12.

• Importance of a Well-Balanced Diet:

• Ensure a diverse and well-balanced diet to cover nutritional needs beyond B12. This promotes overall health and aids in preventing future deficiencies.

B. Vitamin B12 Supplements:

• Oral Supplements:

• Standard treatment often involves oral B12 supplements, typically in the form of cyanocobalamin or methylcobalamin.

• Regular and consistent supplementation is essential, and the dosage is determined by the severity of the deficiency and individual factors.

• Sublingual Supplements:

• Sublingual B12 supplements, which dissolve under the tongue, can enhance absorption and are suitable for individuals with absorption issues.

• This form of supplementation may be preferred by those who have difficulty absorbing B12 through the digestive system.

• Injections for Severe Cases:

• In severe cases or when absorption is severely compromised, B12 injections may be recommended.

• Injections are administered intramuscularly and are particularly effective in rapidly raising B12 levels.

C. Addressing Underlying Causes:

• Intrinsic Factor Deficiency (Pernicious Anemia):

• For individuals with pernicious anemia, lifelong B12 supplementation is necessary.

• Regular monitoring of B12 levels and addressing other associated autoimmune conditions may be part of the management plan.

• Gastrointestinal Conditions:

• Managing underlying gastrointestinal conditions, such as celiac disease or atrophic gastritis, is crucial to improve B12 absorption.

• In some cases, surgical interventions may be considered.

• Medication-Induced Deficiency:

• Adjusting or substituting medications that interfere with B12 absorption, such as proton pump inhibitors or metformin, may be necessary.

• Close monitoring and collaboration with healthcare providers are essential.

Monitoring and Follow-Up:

• Regular monitoring of B12 levels is crucial to assess treatment efficacy and adjust supplementation as needed.

• Periodic health check-ups, including assessments of symptoms and potential side effects, ensure ongoing management and prevention of recurrence.

PREVENTION OF VITAMIN B12 DEFICIENCY

Vitamin B12 deficiency, a condition with diverse health implications, can be effectively prevented through a combination of dietary strategies, targeted supplementation for at-risk groups, and regular health check-ups. This comprehensive approach aims to ensure adequate B12 intake, identify potential risk factors, and intervene proactively to maintain optimal B12 levels.

A. Promoting a Balanced Diet:

• Inclusion of B12-Rich Foods:

• Encourage the consumption of animal products such as meat (beef, pork, lamb), poultry (chicken, turkey), fish (salmon, trout, tuna), dairy products (milk, cheese, yogurt), and eggs.

• Emphasize the importance of a diverse diet to cover nutritional needs beyond B12, fostering overall health.

• Educating Vegetarians and Vegans:

• Provide information on alternative B12 sources for individuals following vegetarian or vegan diets, including fortified foods like certain cereals, plant-based milk, and nutritional yeast.

• Emphasize the importance of monitoring B12 levels and considering supplementation if necessary.

B. Supplementation for At-Risk Groups:

• Vegetarians, Vegans, and Older Adults:

• Consider B12 supplementation for individuals following plant-based diets or those in older age groups with potential absorption issues.

• Sublingual B12 supplements may be suitable for those with absorption challenges.

• Pregnant and Breastfeeding Women:

• Address the increased B12 requirements during pregnancy and breastfeeding through dietary counseling and, if needed, supplementation.

• Promote awareness of potential deficiency symptoms.

C. Regular Health Check-Ups:

• Screening for At-Risk Groups:

• Incorporate B12 screening into routine health check-ups, especially for individuals in high-risk groups such as older people, vegetarians, and those with gastrointestinal conditions.

• Periodic blood tests, including serum B12 levels, help detect deficiency early.

• Evaluation of Symptoms:

• Include questions related to B12 deficiency symptoms in routine medical assessments.

• Recognizing early signs ensures timely intervention and prevents the progression of deficiency.

• Individualized Counseling:

• Provide individualized guidance on B12 needs based on dietary habits, age, and health status.

• Offer advice on supplementation when necessary, tailoring recommendations to each individual's unique circumstances.

CHAPTER TWO

Vitamin B12 Deficiency Diet

Vitamin B12 is essential for various physiological functions, including red blood cell formation, neurological health, and DNA synthesis. A deficiency in this vitamin can lead to a range of health issues, emphasizing the importance of maintaining an adequate intake. Crafting a diet rich in vitamin B12 sources and considering supplementation when necessary is critical to preventing deficiency and supporting overall well-being.

Rich Dietary Sources of Vitamin B12:

• Animal Products: Meat, poultry, fish, dairy, and eggs are primary sources of B12. Include lean meats like beef, pork, poultry and fatty fish like salmon and trout.

• Dairy: Milk, cheese, and yogurt provide B12, offering suitable options for those who include dairy in their diet.

• Eggs: Egg yolks contain B12, making eggs a versatile and nutrient-rich food.

Fortified Foods:

• Plant-Based Options: For individuals following vegetarian or vegan diets, incorporating B12-fortified foods is crucial. Fortified cereals, plant-based milk (soy, almond, rice, or oat milk), and nutritional yeast are viable alternatives.

• Read Labels: Attention food labels, as some processed foods are fortified with B12. Incorporate these fortified options as part of a well-rounded diet.

Supplementation:

• Pills and Sublingual Tablets: B12 supplements are available in various forms, including oral medications and sublingual tablets. These can be convenient for individuals with dietary restrictions or absorption issues.

• Injections: In severe cases or for individuals with significant absorption challenges, B12 injections may be prescribed to ensure rapid and efficient absorption.

Individualized Considerations:

• Tailored Dietary Plans: Work with a healthcare professional or a registered dietitian to create an individualized dietary plan based on lifestyle, preferences, and health conditions.

• Regular Monitoring: Individuals at risk of deficiency, such as vegetarians, older adults, and those with gastrointestinal disorders, should undergo regular health check-ups to monitor B12 levels.

Combining B12 with Other Nutrients:

• Iron and Folate: Ensure an adequate intake of iron and folate, as deficiencies in these nutrients can exacerbate the effects of B12 deficiency. A well-rounded diet with a variety of nutrient-rich foods contributes to overall health.

Dietary Sources of Vitamin B12

Vitamin B12, a crucial nutrient for various bodily functions, is predominantly found in animal products.

Ensuring an adequate intake of B12-rich foods is essential for maintaining optimal health. Let's delve into the diverse dietary sources of Vitamin B12:

Meat and Poultry:

• Beef: Beef, especially organ meats like liver, is an excellent source of B12. Lean cuts of beef provide a substantial amount of this vital nutrient.

• Pork: Pork, including cuts like loin and ham, contains B12. Including a variety of pork products in the diet contributes to overall B12 intake.

• Lamb is another meat source rich in B12, offering a flavorful option for those seeking variety.

Fish and Shellfish:

• Salmon: Fatty fish like salmon are notable for their B12 content. Regular consumption of salmon supports cardiovascular health and provides a significant B12 boost.

• Trout: Trout, a freshwater fish, is a nutritious option for B12. Grilled or baked trout can be incorporated into a balanced diet.

• Tuna: Whether fresh or canned, tuna is a versatile and accessible source of B12. It can be included in salads, sandwiches, or as a main dish.

• Shellfish: Clams, mussels, crabs, and other shellfish are rich in B12. These seafood options offer a tasty and nutrient-dense addition to the diet.

Dairy Products:

• Milk: Cow's milk is fortified with B12 and serves as a reliable source of this nutrient. Whether consumed on its own or incorporated into various recipes, milk contributes to B12 intake.

• Cheese: Various types of cheese, including cheddar, Swiss, and mozzarella, contain B12. Cheese is a versatile ingredient that adds flavor to many dishes.

• Yogurt: Yogurt is nutritious, particularly in varieties with added B12. It can be enjoyed as a snack or as part of a meal.

Eggs:

• Whole Eggs: Eggs, specifically the yolk, are rich in B12. Incorporating eggs into the diet provides a wholesome and complete source of various essential nutrients.

• Egg Dishes: Dishes like omelets, frittatas, and scrambled eggs offer tasty ways to include B12 in meals.

Considerations for Dietary Choices:

• Variety is Key: Including a variety of B12-rich foods ensures a diverse nutrient profile and helps meet overall dietary needs.

• Cooking Methods: While cooking methods like grilling, baking, and boiling preserve B12 content, prolonged cooking or high heat can lead to nutrient loss.

CHALLENGES FOR INDIVIDUALS WITH DIETARY RESTRICTIONS

Maintaining optimal Vitamin B12 levels can pose challenges for individuals with dietary restrictions, particularly vegetarians and vegans. These nutritional choices may limit the natural sources of B12, which are predominantly found in animal products. However, with awareness and strategic dietary planning, individuals can overcome these challenges and ensure sufficient B12 intake.

Vegetarians:

• Challenge: While vegetarians include dairy and eggs in their diet, the primary sources of B12 still need to be improved compared to those who consume meat.

• Strategies:

• Incorporate Dairy Products: Regular consumption of dairy products such as milk, yogurt, and cheese can contribute to B12 intake.

• Eggs as a Source: Including eggs in various forms, such

as boiled, scrambled, or as part of dishes, provides B12.

• Variety in Plant-Based Foods: Incorporate B12-fortified plant-based foods to diversify nutrient intake.

Vegans:

• Challenge: Vegans, who exclude all animal products from their diet, face a more significant challenge in obtaining B12 naturally.

• Strategies:

• Fortified Foods: Rely on B12-fortified foods to bridge the nutrient gap. This includes fortified plant-based milk, cereals, and nutritional yeast.

• Supplementation: Consider B12 supplements to ensure adequate intake, especially for individuals who may find it challenging to meet their B12 needs solely through diet.

C. Fortified Foods:

• Challenge: While fortified foods offer a valuable solution, their availability and the level of fortification can vary.

• Strategies:

• Fortified Cereals: Choose cereals that are fortified explicitly with B12. These can be a convenient and tasty way to incorporate the vitamin into the diet.

• Plant-Based Milk: Opt for plant-based milk alternatives, like soy, almond, or oat milk, that are fortified with B12. These options provide a dairy-free alternative while still contributing to B12 intake.

• Nutritional Yeast: This yeast product is often used in vegan cooking for its cheesy flavor. It can be sprinkled on dishes or incorporated into recipes, providing a source of B12.

Considerations for Effective B12 Intake:

• Label Reading: Pay attention to food labels to identify B12-fortified products and determine the amount of B12 provided.

• Diverse Food Choices: Incorporate a variety of B12-rich foods, both natural and fortified, to ensure a well-rounded nutrient intake.

• Supplementation Guidance: Consult with healthcare professionals to determine the need for B12 supplements and establish the appropriate dosage.

THE IMPORTANCE OF FOLLOWING A VITAMIN B12 DEFICIENCY DIET AS A PATIENT

For individuals diagnosed with Vitamin B12 deficiency, adopting and adhering to a B12 deficiency diet is crucial for managing symptoms, preventing complications, and promoting overall well-being. Understanding the significance of dietary modifications and the role of specific foods is essential in effectively addressing B12 deficiency.

Symptom Management:

• Neurological Health: Vitamin B12 is vital for neurological function. Following a B12-rich diet helps alleviate symptoms such as numbness, tingling, difficulty walking, and cognitive disturbances associated with neurological deficiency complications.

• Fatigue and Anemia: Adequate B12 intake supports the production of healthy red blood cells, addressing fatigue and preventing or treating anemia associated with B12 deficiency.

Prevention of Complications:

• Cognitive Impairment: B12 deficiency has been linked to cognitive decline and memory disturbances. By following a B12 deficiency diet, patients aim to mitigate the risk of long-term cognitive complications.

• Neuropathy: Peripheral neuropathy, characterized by nerve damage leading to numbness and

Promoting Recovery:

• Optimal Absorption: A well-planned B12 deficiency diet not only includes B12-rich foods but also considers factors that enhance B12 absorption. This can aid in a quicker recovery and improvement of B12 levels.

• Comprehensive Nutrient Intake: Following a B12 deficiency diet ensures not only sufficient B12 but also a diverse intake of other essential nutrients, contributing to overall health.

Lifestyle Adaptations:

• Dietary Choices: Patients learn to make informed nutritional choices, incorporating B12-rich sources such as meats, fish, dairy, and eggs. Awareness of fortified foods and possible supplementation becomes crucial for vegetarians or vegans.

• Meal Planning: Adopting a B12 deficiency diet involves thoughtful meal planning to achieve a balance of nutrients. Consulting with a dietitian can provide personalized guidance.

Monitoring and Adjustment:

• Regular Check-Ups: Patients following a B12 deficiency

diet should undergo regular check-ups to monitor B12 levels and assess the effectiveness of dietary changes.

• Supplementation Guidance: Healthcare professionals sometimes may recommend B12 supplements to complement dietary intake. Compliance with supplementation guidelines is integral to achieving optimal B12 levels.

Quality of Life Improvement:

• Energy Levels: Addressing B12 deficiency through diet positively impacts energy levels, reducing fatigue and enhancing the overall quality of life.

• Mental Well-Being: Improved neurological function contributes to better mental well-being, enhancing mood and cognitive performance.

VITAMIN B12 DEFICIENCY DIET MEAL PLANS

Vitamin B12 deficiency can significantly impact overall health and well-being, but proper dietary planning can meet your nutritional needs and mitigate the effects of deficiency. Here are several well-balanced meal plans designed to address Vitamin B12 deficiency over the course of Ten days:

DAY 1:

Breakfast:

- Fortified whole grain cereal with fortified almond milk

- Mixed berries on top

- Whole grain toast with avocado

Lunch:

- Chickpea and spinach curry served with brown rice

- Side salad with mixed greens, cherry tomatoes, and balsamic vinaigrette

Dinner:

- Grilled tofu with roasted vegetables (bell peppers, zucchini, and carrots)

- Quinoa pilaf with chopped parsley

DAY 2:

Breakfast:

• Vegan fortified breakfast burrito with tofu scramble, black beans, spinach, and avocado wrapped in a whole wheat tortilla.

• Fresh fruit salad on the side

Lunch:

• Lentil soup with vegetables (carrots, celery, and onions)

• Whole grain roll with vegan butter

• Mixed green salad with chickpeas and tahini dressing

Dinner:

• Baked cod with herbed breadcrumbs

• Steamed broccoli and cauliflower

• Quinoa and black bean salad with cilantro lime dressing

DAY 3:

Breakfast:

• Fortified almond milk chia pudding with fresh berries and sliced almonds

• Whole grain toast with almond butter

Lunch:

• Vegan fortified nutritional yeast pasta with marinara sauce, sautéed mushrooms, and spinach

• Mixed green salad with walnuts, dried cranberries, and balsamic vinaigrette

Dinner:

• Vegetable stir-fry with tofu, bell peppers, snap peas, and broccoli served over brown rice

• Steamed edamame on the side

DAY 4:

Breakfast:

• Vegan fortified smoothie bowl made with fortified plant-based milk, spinach, banana, and chia seeds and topped with granola, sliced banana, and coconut flakes.

Lunch:

• Quinoa and black bean bowl with roasted sweet potatoes, avocado, cherry tomatoes, and lime tahini dressing

Dinner:

• Vegan chickpea and spinach curry served with quinoa

• Side of steamed green beans with lemon zest

DAY 5:

Breakfast:

• Vegan fortified almond milk oatmeal topped with mixed berries, chopped nuts, and a drizzle of maple syrup

• Whole grain toast with mashed avocado and sliced tomato

Lunch:

• Vegan lentil salad with mixed greens, roasted beets, carrots, and lemon-tahini dressing

• Whole grain roll with hummus

Dinner:

• Vegan fortified nutritional yeast pasta with roasted cherry tomatoes, garlic, and basil

• Steamed asparagus with lemon zest

DAY 6:

Breakfast:

• Vegan fortified almond milk smoothie with spinach, banana, frozen mixed berries, and a scoop of vegan protein powder

• Whole grain toast with almond butter and sliced strawberries

Lunch:

• Vegan lentil soup with diced carrots, celery, and onions

• Whole grain crackers with hummus

• Side salad with mixed greens, cucumber, and lemon-tahini dressing

Dinner:

• Vegan tofu and vegetable stir-fry with bell peppers, broccoli, snap peas, and a tangy soy-ginger sauce served over brown rice.

• Steamed bok choy with sesame seeds

DAY 7:

Breakfast:

• Fortified whole grain cereal with fortified oat milk

• Sliced banana and chopped walnuts on top

• Whole grain English muffin with mashed avocado and tomato slices

Lunch:

• Vegan black bean and sweet potato salad with diced bell peppers, corn, red onion, and cilantro-lime vinaigrette

• Whole grain roll with vegan butter

Dinner:

• Vegan chickpea and spinach curry served with quinoa

• Steamed broccoli with lemon zest

• Side of naan bread

DAY 8:

Breakfast:

• Vegan fortified almond milk yogurt parfait with layers of granola, mixed berries, and sliced almonds

• Whole grain toast with almond butter and sliced banana

Lunch:

• Vegan Mediterranean quinoa salad with diced cucumber, cherry tomatoes, Kalamata olives, red onion, and lemon-tahini dressing

• Whole grain pita bread with hummus

Dinner:

• Vegan fortified nutritional yeast pasta with roasted cherry tomatoes, garlic, and basil

• Side of steamed green beans with almond slices

DAY 9:

Breakfast:

• Vegan fortified smoothie bowl made with fortified plant-based milk, kale, pineapple, and banana, topped with granola, shredded coconut, and chia seeds

Lunch:

• Vegan avocado and white bean wrap with shredded carrots, cucumber, mixed greens, and a creamy tahini dressing, wrapped in a whole wheat tortilla

• Side of carrot sticks with hummus

Dinner:

• Vegan lentil and vegetable stew served with crusty whole-grain bread

• Side salad with mixed greens, cherry tomatoes, and balsamic vinaigrette

DAY 10:

Breakfast:

• Fortified almond milk chia pudding with fresh mango chunks and toasted coconut flakes

• Whole grain toast with mashed avocado and sliced tomato

Lunch:

• Vegan quinoa and black bean burrito bowl with roasted sweet potatoes, avocado, cherry tomatoes, and lime-tahini dressing

Dinner:

• Vegan tofu and vegetable curry with coconut milk served over brown rice

• Steamed snow peas with sesame seeds

CHAPTER THREE

Meat and Poultry Recipes

Grilled Lemon and Herb Chicken Breast

Meal Description: Enjoy a delightful and healthy meal with our Grilled Lemon and Herb Chicken Breast. This flavorful dish combines the zesty freshness of lemon with aromatic herbs to create a light, satisfying, and low-calorie option. Perfect for a quick and easy weeknight dinner or a weekend barbecue.

Ingredients:

• Four boneless, skinless chicken breasts

• Two lemons (juiced and zested)

• Three tablespoons olive oil

• Two cloves garlic, minced

• One teaspoon dried oregano

• One teaspoon dried thyme

• Salt and black pepper to taste

• Fresh parsley for garnish (optional)

Instructions:

• Marinate the Chicken:

• Combine lemon juice, lemon zest, olive oil, minced garlic, dried oregano, dried thyme, salt, and black pepper in a bowl. Mix well to create the marinade.

• Place the chicken breasts in a resealable plastic bag or shallow dish and pour half of the marinade over them. Ensure the chicken is evenly coated. Marinate in the refrigerator for at least 30 minutes.

• Preheat the Grill:

• Preheat your grill to medium-high heat.

• Grill the Chicken:

• Remove the chicken from the marinade, allowing any excess to drip off. Discard the used marinade.

• Place the chicken breasts on the preheated grill. Grill for approximately 6-8 minutes per side or until the internal temperature reaches 165°F (74°C) and the chicken is cooked through.

• Baste the chicken with the remaining marinade during the last few minutes of grilling for an extra burst of flavor.

• Serve:

• Once cooked, transfer the grilled chicken to a serving platter.

• Garnish with fresh parsley if desired.

Nutrition Information (Per Serving):

• Calories: 220

• Protein: 30g

• Carbohydrates: 3g

• Fat: 10g

• Saturated Fat: 1.5g

• Cholesterol: 80mg

• Sodium: 300mg

• Fiber: 1g

• Sugar: 1g

BEEF STIR-FRY WITH VEGETABLES

Meal Description: Indulge in a delicious and wholesome Beef Stir-Fry with Vegetables—a quick and flavorful dish that brings together tender beef strips and an array of colorful vegetables. This stir-fry is satisfying and a perfect balance of protein and veggies for a nutritious meal.

Ingredients:

• 1 lb (450g) sirloin or flank steak, thinly sliced

• Two tablespoons of soy sauce

• One tablespoon of oyster sauce

• One tablespoon of hoisin sauce

• One tablespoon cornstarch

• Two tablespoons vegetable oil divided

• Three cloves garlic, minced

• One tablespoon ginger, grated

• One bell pepper, thinly sliced

• 1 cup broccoli florets

• One carrot, julienned

• 1 cup snap peas, ends trimmed

• Two green onions, sliced

• Sesame seeds for garnish (optional)

• Cooked brown rice or noodles for serving

Instructions:

• Prepare the Marinade:

• Combine soy sauce, oyster sauce, hoisin sauce, and cornstarch in a bowl. Mix until the cornstarch is fully dissolved.

• Add the thinly sliced beef to the marinade, ensuring each piece is well-coated. Let it marinate for at least 15 minutes.

• Stir-Fry the Beef:

• Heat one tablespoon of vegetable oil in a wok or large skillet over high heat.

• Add the marinated beef to the hot pan, spreading it out to ensure even cooking. Stir-fry for 2-3 minutes or until the beef is browned and cooked through. Remove the meat from the pan and set it aside.

• Cook the Vegetables:

• In the same pan, add another tablespoon of oil if needed.

• Add minced garlic and grated ginger, sautéing for about 30 seconds until fragrant.

• Add the bell pepper, broccoli, carrot, and snap peas to the pan. Stir-fry the vegetables for 3-4 minutes or until they are tender-crisp.

• Combine and Finish:

• Return the cooked beef to the pan with the vegetables.

• Add sliced green onions and toss everything together

until well combined and heated through.

• Adjust seasoning if necessary and sprinkle with sesame seeds for garnish if desired.

• Serve:

• Serve the Beef Stir-Fry over cooked brown rice or noodles.

Nutrition Information (Per Serving, excluding rice/noodles):

• Calories: 350

• Protein: 30g

• Carbohydrates: 18g

• Fat: 18g

• Saturated Fat: 4g

• Cholesterol: 70mg

• Sodium: 800mg

• Fiber: 4g

• Sugar: 6g

BAKED TURKEY MEATBALLS

Meal Description: Savor lean protein goodness with these delicious Baked Turkey Meatballs. These tender and flavorful meatballs are baked to perfection, offering a healthier alternative without compromising on taste. It is ideal for pairing with pasta, salads, or as a delightful appetizer.

Ingredients:

- 1 lb (450g) ground turkey

- 1/2 cup breadcrumbs (whole wheat for a healthier option)

- 1/4 cup grated Parmesan cheese

- 1/4 cup fresh parsley, finely chopped

- 1/4 cup onion, finely minced

- Two cloves garlic, minced

- One large egg

- One teaspoon dried oregano

- One teaspoon of dried basil

- 1/2 teaspoon salt

- 1/4 teaspoon black pepper

• Olive oil spray

Instructions:

• Preheat the Oven:

• Preheat your oven to 375°F (190°C). Line a baking sheet with parchment paper or lightly grease it.

• Prepare the Meatball Mixture:

• In a large mixing bowl, combine ground turkey, breadcrumbs, grated Parmesan cheese, chopped parsley, minced onion, minced garlic, egg, oregano, basil, salt, and black pepper.

• Gently mix the ingredients until well combined. Avoid overmixing to keep the meatballs tender.

• Shape the Meatballs:

• With clean hands, scoop out portions of the mixture and roll them into meatballs, each about 1 inch in diameter. Place the meatballs on the prepared baking sheet, leaving some space between each.

• Bake the Meatballs:

• Lightly spray the tops of the meatballs with olive oil spray. This helps them brown nicely in the oven.

• Bake in the preheated oven for 20-25 minutes or until the meatballs are cooked through and browned on the outside.

• Serve and Enjoy:

• Once baked, remove the meatballs from the oven and let them rest for a few minutes.

• Serve the turkey meatballs as desired, whether over pasta, in a sub sandwich, or as an appetizer.

Nutrition Information (Per Serving):

- Calories: 160

- Protein: 20g

- Carbohydrates: 7g

- Fat: 6g

- Saturated Fat: 2g

- Cholesterol: 80mg

- Sodium: 350mg

- Fiber: 1g

- Sugar: 1g

LAMB KEBABS WITH MINT YOGURT SAUCE

Meal Description: Transport your taste buds to the Mediterranean with these succulent Lamb Kebabs paired with a refreshing Mint Yogurt Sauce. The aromatic blend of spices in the lamb and the coolness of the mint-infused yogurt create a delightful dish perfect for a barbecue, family dinner, or special occasion.

Ingredients:

For Lamb Kebabs:

- 1.5 lbs (680g) ground lamb

- One small onion, finely grated

- Three cloves garlic, minced

- One teaspoon of ground cumin

- One teaspoon of ground coriander

- One teaspoon paprika

- 1/2 teaspoon ground cinnamon

- Salt and black pepper to taste

- Wooden skewers soaked in water

For Mint Yogurt Sauce:

• 1 cup Greek yogurt

• 1/4 cup fresh mint leaves, finely chopped

• One tablespoon of lemon juice

• One teaspoon honey

• Salt to taste

Instructions:

• Prepare the Lamb Kebab Mixture:

• Combine ground lamb, grated onion, minced garlic, cumin, coriander, paprika, cinnamon, salt, and black pepper in a large bowl. Mix well until the spices are evenly distributed.

• Shape the Kebabs:

• Take a handful of the lamb mixture and mold it onto a wooden skewer, forming a kebab shape. Repeat until all the mixture is used.

• Place the skewers on a plate and refrigerate for at least 30 minutes to allow the flavors to meld.

• Preheat the Grill:

• Preheat your grill or grill pan to medium-high heat.

• Grill the Lamb Kebabs:

• Lightly oil the grill grates or grill pan to prevent sticking.

• Grill the lamb kebabs for approximately 4-5 minutes per side or until they reach your desired level of doneness.

• Prepare the Mint Yogurt Sauce:

• Combine Greek yogurt, chopped mint, lemon juice, honey, and salt in a small bowl. Mix thoroughly to create the mint yogurt sauce.

• Serve:

• Arrange the grilled lamb kebabs on a serving platter.

• Serve the kebabs with a side of Mint Yogurt Sauce for dipping.

Nutrition Information (Per Serving, excluding sauce):

• Calories: 280

• Protein: 20g

• Carbohydrates: 2g

• Fat: 22g

• Saturated Fat: 10g

• Cholesterol: 90mg

• Sodium: 80mg

• Fiber: 0g

• Sugar: 0g

PORK TENDERLOIN WITH APPLE CHUTNEY

Meal Description: Indulge in a delightful blend of savory and sweet with this Pork Tenderloin accompanied by Apple Chutney. The succulent and juicy pork pairs perfectly with the warm and spiced apple chutney, creating a comforting dish that's perfect for a cozy dinner or a special gathering.

Ingredients:

For Pork Tenderloin:

• Two pork tenderloins (about 1.5 lbs each)

• Two tablespoons of olive oil

• Two teaspoons of dried thyme

• Salt and black pepper to taste

For Apple Chutney:

• Two apples, peeled, cored, and diced (use a sweet variety like Fuji or Honeycrisp)

• 1/2 cup red onion, finely chopped

• 1/4 cup brown sugar

• 1/4 cup apple cider vinegar

- One teaspoon ground cinnamon

- 1/2 teaspoon ground ginger

- 1/4 teaspoon ground cloves

- Salt to taste

Instructions:

- Preheat the Oven:

- Preheat your oven to 375°F (190°C).

- Prepare the Pork Tenderloin:

- Pat the pork tenderloins dry with paper towels.

- Mix olive oil, dried thyme, salt, and black pepper in a small bowl to create a marinade.

- Rub the pork tenderloins with the marinade, ensuring they are well-coated.

- Sear the Pork:

- Heat an oven-safe skillet over medium-high heat. Sear the pork tenderloins on all sides until they develop a golden-brown crust.

- Roast in the Oven:

- Transfer the skillet to the preheated oven and roast the pork for about 20-25 minutes or until the internal temperature reaches 145°F (63°C). Cooking time may vary based on the thickness of the tenderloins.

- Prepare the Apple Chutney:

- In a saucepan, combine diced apples, chopped red onion, brown sugar, apple cider vinegar, ground cinnamon, ground ginger, ground cloves, and a pinch of salt.

- Simmer over medium heat, stirring occasionally, until

the apples are soft and the chutney has thickened. This usually takes about 15-20 minutes.

• Slice and Serve:

• Allow the pork tenderloins to rest for a few minutes before slicing.

• Serve the sliced pork with a generous spoonful of warm apple chutney on top.

Nutrition Information (Per Serving, including chutney):

• Calories: 300

• Protein: 25g

• Carbohydrates: 20g

• Fat: 12g

• Saturated Fat: 3g

• Cholesterol: 75mg

• Sodium: 300mg

• Fiber: 3g

• Sugar: 15g

CHICKEN AND BROCCOLI CASSEROLE

Meal Description: Savor the comforting flavors of a classic Chicken and Broccoli Casserole. This hearty and wholesome dish combines tender chicken, crisp broccoli, and a creamy sauce topped with a golden layer of melted cheese. Perfect for a family dinner or potluck gathering, this casserole is sure to become a favorite.

Ingredients:

For the Casserole:

- 4 cups cooked chicken breast, shredded

- 4 cups broccoli florets, blanched

- 2 cups shredded cheddar cheese

- 1 cup mayonnaise

- 1 cup sour cream

- 1 cup chicken broth

- 1/2 cup grated Parmesan cheese

- Three tablespoons of all-purpose flour

- Two tablespoons unsalted butter

- Two teaspoons of Dijon mustard

- Two cloves garlic, minced

- Salt and black pepper to taste

For Topping:

- 1 cup breadcrumbs

- Two tablespoons melted butter

- 1/4 cup chopped fresh parsley (optional)

Instructions:

- Preheat the Oven:

- Preheat your oven to 375°F (190°C).

- Prepare the Chicken and Broccoli:

- In a large mixing bowl, combine the shredded chicken and blanched broccoli. Set aside.

- Make the Sauce:

- In a saucepan over medium heat, melt the butter. Add minced garlic and cook until fragrant.

- Whisk in the flour to create a roux. Cook for 1-2 minutes, stirring continuously.

- Gradually add the chicken broth, mayonnaise, sour cream, Dijon mustard, salt, and black pepper. Continue whisking until the sauce thickens.

- Stir in the shredded cheddar cheese and grated Parmesan until melted and smooth.

- Combine Sauce with Chicken and Broccoli:

- Pour the cheese sauce over the chicken and broccoli mixture. Gently fold until the ingredients are evenly coated.

- Prepare the Topping:

- In a small bowl, mix breadcrumbs with melted butter.

- Assemble and Bake:

- Transfer the chicken and broccoli mixture into a greased casserole dish.

- Sprinkle the breadcrumb topping evenly over the casserole.

- Bake in the Oven:

- Bake in the preheated oven for 25-30 minutes or until the casserole is bubbly and the top is golden brown.

- Serve:

- Remove from the oven and let it rest for a few minutes.

- Garnish with chopped fresh parsley if desired.

- Serve the Chicken and Broccoli Casserole warm, and enjoy!

Nutrition Information (Per Serving):

- Calories: 400

- Protein: 25g

- Carbohydrates: 15g

- Fat: 28g

- Saturated Fat: 12g

- Cholesterol: 85mg

- Sodium: 600mg

- Fiber: 2g

- Sugar: 3g

SPICY TURKEY CHILI

Meal Description: Warm up your taste buds with a hearty and flavorful Spicy Turkey Chili bowl. Packed with lean ground turkey, beans, and a medley of spices, this chili combines comfort and kick perfectly. Whether you're feeding a crowd or enjoying a cozy night in, this chili will satisfy your cravings for a bold and spicy meal.

Ingredients:

• 1.5 lbs (680g) ground turkey

• One large onion, diced

• Three cloves garlic, minced

• One red bell pepper, diced

• One green bell pepper, diced

• One jalapeño pepper, finely chopped (seeds removed for less heat, if desired)

• Two cans (15 oz each) of kidney beans, drained and rinsed

• One can (15 oz) black beans, drained and rinsed

• One can (28 oz) crushed tomatoes

• 1 cup low-sodium chicken broth

• Two tablespoons of tomato paste

• Two teaspoons of chili powder

- One teaspoon of ground cumin

- One teaspoon of smoked paprika

- 1/2 teaspoon cayenne pepper (adjust for desired spice level)

- Salt and black pepper to taste

- Olive oil for cooking

- Optional toppings: shredded cheddar cheese, chopped green onions, sour cream, cilantro

Instructions:

- Sauté Aromatics:

- Heat olive oil over medium heat in a large pot or Dutch oven. Add diced onion, minced garlic, and chopped jalapeño. Sauté until the onions are translucent.

- Brown the Turkey:

- Add ground turkey to the pot. Break it apart with a spoon and cook until browned.

- Add Vegetables:

- Stir in diced red and green bell peppers. Cook for 3-4 minutes until the peppers begin to soften.

- Season the Chili:

- Add chili powder, ground cumin, smoked paprika, cayenne pepper, salt, and black pepper. Stir well to coat the meat and vegetables with the spices.

- Incorporate Beans and Tomatoes:

- Pour in drained and rinsed kidney beans and black beans. Add crushed tomatoes, chicken broth, and tomato paste. Stir to combine.

• Simmer:

• Bring the chili to a simmer. Reduce the heat to low, cover the pot, and let it simmer for at least 30 minutes to allow the flavors to meld. Stir occasionally.

• Adjust Seasoning:

• Taste the chili and adjust the seasoning if needed. Add more chili powder or cayenne pepper for extra heat.

• Serve:

• Ladle the Spicy Turkey Chili into bowls. If desired, top with shredded cheddar cheese, chopped green onions, sour cream, or cilantro.

Nutrition Information (Per Serving, without toppings):

• Calories: 350

• Protein: 30g

• Carbohydrates: 30g

• Fat: 12g

• Saturated Fat: 3g

• Cholesterol: 70mg

• Sodium: 600mg

• Fiber: 10g

• Sugar: 5g

HONEY MUSTARD GLAZED SALMON

Meal Description: Elevate your seafood dinner with the delightful combination of sweet and tangy flavors in this Honey Mustard Glazed Salmon. This quick and easy recipe transforms salmon fillets into a mouthwatering dish that's perfect for a weeknight dinner or a special occasion. Serve it with your favorite sides for a wholesome and delicious meal.

Ingredients:

• Four salmon fillets (about 6 oz each), skin-on

• 1/4 cup Dijon mustard

• Two tablespoons honey

• Two tablespoons of whole-grain mustard

• One tablespoon of soy sauce

• Two cloves garlic, minced

• One tablespoon of olive oil

• Salt and black pepper to taste

• Fresh lemon wedges for serving

• Chopped fresh parsley for garnish (optional)

Instructions:

- Preheat the Oven:

- Preheat your oven to 400°F (200°C).

- Prepare the Honey Mustard Glaze:

- Whisk together Dijon mustard, honey, whole grain mustard, soy sauce, minced garlic, olive oil, salt, and black pepper in a small bowl. Ensure the glaze is well combined.

- Marinate the Salmon:

- Place the salmon fillets, skin-side down, in a baking dish or on a lined baking sheet.

- Brush the honey mustard glaze generously over the salmon fillets, ensuring an even coating.

- Bake in the Oven:

- Bake the salmon in the preheated oven for 12-15 minutes or until the salmon is cooked through and flakes easily with a fork. Cooking time may vary based on the thickness of the fillets.

- Broil for a Crispy Top (Optional):

- If you desire a slightly crispy top, switch the oven to broil for the last 2-3 minutes, keeping a close eye to prevent burning.

- Serve:

- Remove the salmon from the oven and let it rest for a few minutes.

- Serve the Honey Mustard Glazed Salmon over your favorite grains or alongside roasted vegetables.

- Garnish with chopped fresh parsley and lemon wedges for an extra burst of freshness.

Nutrition Information (Per Serving):

- Calories: 350

- Protein: 30g

- Carbohydrates: 12g

- Fat: 18g

- Saturated Fat: 3g

- Cholesterol: 80mg

- Sodium: 500mg

- Fiber: 1g

- Sugar: 9g

CHAPTER FOUR

Fish and Shellfish Recipes

Baked Lemon Garlic Salmon

Meal Description: Experience the vibrant and zesty flavors of Baked Lemon Garlic Salmon, a simple yet elegant dish showcasing fresh salmon's natural goodness. This recipe combines the brightness of lemon, the richness of garlic, and the tenderness of baked salmon for a delicious and wholesome meal.

Ingredients:

• Four salmon fillets (about 6 oz each), skin-on

• Three tablespoons olive oil

• Four cloves garlic, minced

• Zest of 1 lemon

• Juice of 1 lemon

• One teaspoon dried oregano

• One teaspoon of dried thyme

• Salt and black pepper to taste

• Lemon slices for garnish

• Fresh parsley, chopped, for garnish

Instructions:

• Preheat the Oven:

• Preheat your oven to 400°F (200°C).

• Prepare the Lemon Garlic Marinade:

• In a small bowl, combine olive oil, minced garlic, lemon zest, lemon juice, dried oregano, dried thyme, salt, and black pepper. Mix well to create the marinade.

• Marinate the Salmon:

• Place the salmon fillets, skin-side down, in a baking dish or on a lined baking sheet.

• Brush the lemon garlic marinade generously over the salmon fillets, ensuring an even coating.

• Bake in the Oven:

• Bake the salmon in the preheated oven for 12-15 minutes or until the salmon is cooked through and flakes easily with a fork. Cooking time may vary based on the thickness of the fillets.

• Broil for a Golden Top (Optional):

• If you desire a golden top, switch the oven to broil for the last 2-3 minutes, keeping a close eye to prevent burning.

• Serve:

• Remove the salmon from the oven and let it rest for a few minutes.

• Garnish with fresh lemon slices and chopped parsley.

• Serve the Baked Lemon Garlic Salmon over your favorite grains or alongside steamed vegetables.

Nutrition Information (Per Serving):

• Calories: 350

• Protein: 30g

• Carbohydrates: 2g

• Fat: 24g

• Saturated Fat: 4g

• Cholesterol: 80mg

• Sodium: 200mg

- Fiber: 1g
- Sugar: 0g

SHRIMP SCAMPI WITH LINGUINE

Meal Description: Indulge in the classic and delectable flavors of Shrimp Scampi with Linguine. This dish features succulent shrimp cooked in a flavorful garlic and white wine sauce, served over linguine pasta. With a perfect balance of zesty citrus and savory goodness, this shrimp scampi is a delightful choice for an elegant dinner.

Ingredients:

• 1 lb (450g) linguine pasta

• 1.5 lbs (680g) large shrimp, peeled and deveined

• Four tablespoons unsalted butter

• Four tablespoons of olive oil

• Five cloves garlic, minced

• 1/2 teaspoon red pepper flakes (adjust to taste)

• Zest of 1 lemon

• Juice of 1 lemon

• 1/2 cup dry white wine

• Salt and black pepper to taste

• Fresh parsley, chopped, for garnish

• Grated Parmesan cheese for serving

Instructions:

• Cook the Linguine:

• Cook the linguine pasta in a large pot of salted boiling water according to the package instructions until al dente. Drain and set aside.

• Prepare the Shrimp:

• Pat the shrimp dry with paper towels and season with salt and black pepper.

• Sauté the Shrimp:

• Heat 2 tablespoons of butter and two tablespoons of olive oil over medium-high heat in a large skillet or pan.

• Add the seasoned shrimp to the skillet and cook for 1-2 minutes on each side or until they turn pink and opaque. Remove the shrimp from the pan and set aside.

• Make the Scampi Sauce:

• Add the remaining two tablespoons of butter and two tablespoons of olive oil in the same skillet.

• Sauté minced garlic and red pepper flakes until fragrant (about 1 minute).

• Pour in the white wine, lemon zest, and lemon juice. Bring to a simmer and let it cook for 2-3 minutes.

• Combine Shrimp and Linguine:

• Return the cooked shrimp to the skillet, tossing them in the scampi sauce to coat evenly.

• Serve:

• Serve the Shrimp Scampi over a bed of cooked linguine.

• Garnish with chopped fresh parsley and grated Parmesan cheese.

Nutrition Information (Per Serving):

• Calories: 500

• Protein: 30g

• Carbohydrates: 50g

• Fat: 20g

• Saturated Fat: 8g

• Cholesterol: 180mg

• Sodium: 400mg

• Fiber: 3g

• Sugar: 2g

TUNA NIÇOISE SALAD

Meal Description: Experience the vibrant flavors of the Mediterranean with Tuna Niçoise Salad—a classic French dish that combines the richness of tuna, the freshness of vegetables, and the saltiness of olives and capers. This hearty salad is delicious and nutritious for a satisfying lunch or dinner.

Ingredients:

For the Salad:

• 1 lb (450g) small new potatoes, halved

• Four large eggs

• 8 oz (225g) green beans, trimmed

• 1 cup cherry tomatoes, halved

• 1 cup Niçoise olives

• 4 cups mixed salad greens (e.g., arugula, spinach, or butter lettuce)

For the Tuna:

• Two cans (5 oz each) of tuna in olive oil, drained

• Salt and black pepper to taste

• One tablespoon of lemon juice

• One tablespoon extra-virgin olive oil

For the Dressing:

• Three tablespoons of red wine vinegar

• One teaspoon of Dijon mustard

• One clove of garlic, minced

• 1/2 cup extra-virgin olive oil

• Salt and black pepper to taste

Optional Garnish:

• Fresh parsley, chopped

• Capers

Instructions:

• Prepare the Potatoes:

• Boil the halved new potatoes in salted water until fork-tender. Drain and set aside.

• Boil the Eggs:

• Place the eggs in a saucepan and cover with water. Bring to a boil, then reduce heat and simmer for 9-10 minutes. Transfer the eggs to an ice bath to cool. Once cooled, peel and halve them.

• Blanch the Green Beans:

• Blanch the green beans in boiling salted water for 2-3 minutes until they are crisp-tender. Transfer to an ice bath to stop the cooking process.

• Prepare the Tuna:

• Combine drained tuna, salt, black pepper, lemon juice, and olive oil in a bowl. Gently flake the tuna with a fork.

• Assemble the Salad:

• Arrange the salad greens on a platter. Top with boiled potatoes, blanched green beans, cherry tomatoes, olives, halved eggs, and the seasoned tuna.

• Make the Dressing:

• Whisk together red wine vinegar, Dijon mustard, minced garlic, salt, and black pepper in a small bowl. Slowly drizzle in the olive oil while whisking until the dressing emulsifies.

• Drizzle with Dressing:

• Drizzle the dressing over the salad just before serving.

• Garnish and Serve:

• Garnish with fresh parsley and capers if desired.

• Serve the Tuna Niçoise Salad immediately, offering extra dressing on the side.

Nutrition Information (Per Serving):

• Calories: 400

• Protein: 20g

• Carbohydrates: 30g

• Fat: 25g

• Saturated Fat: 4g

• Cholesterol: 140mg

• Sodium: 600mg

• Fiber: 6g

• Sugar: 4g

GRILLED HALIBUT WITH MANGO SALSA

Meal Description: Indulge in the perfect blend of flavors with Grilled Halibut topped with vibrant Mango Salsa. This light and refreshing dish brings together the mildness of halibut and the sweet-tangy goodness of mango salsa. Ideal for a summer barbecue or a quick and healthy dinner, this recipe is a feast for the senses.

Ingredients:

For the Grilled Halibut:

• Four halibut fillets (6 oz each)

• Two tablespoons of olive oil

• One teaspoon paprika

• One teaspoon of garlic powder

• Salt and black pepper to taste

• Fresh lemon wedges for serving

For the Mango Salsa:

• Two ripe mangoes, peeled, pitted, and diced

• One red bell pepper, diced

- 1/2 red onion, finely chopped

- One jalapeño, seeded and finely chopped

- 1/4 cup fresh cilantro, chopped

- Juice of 2 limes

- Salt and black pepper to taste

Instructions:

- Prepare the Grilled Halibut:

- Preheat the grill to medium-high heat.

- Pat the halibut fillets dry with paper towels.

- Mix a marinade with olive oil, paprika, garlic powder, salt, and black pepper in a small bowl.

- Brush the halibut fillets with the marinade, ensuring they are well-coated.

- Grill the Halibut:

- Place the halibut fillets on the preheated grill. Grill for 3-4 minutes per side or until the fish is opaque and flakes easily with a fork.

- Prepare the Mango Salsa:

- Combine diced mangoes, red bell pepper, red onion, jalapeño, cilantro, lime juice, salt, and black pepper in a mixing bowl. Mix well to combine.

- Serve:

- Transfer the grilled halibut fillets to serving plates.

- Spoon the mango salsa over the top of each fillet.

- Garnish with additional cilantro and serve with fresh lemon wedges.

Nutrition Information (Per Serving):

- Calories: 300
- Protein: 30g
- Carbohydrates: 20g
- Fat: 12g
- Saturated Fat: 2g
- Cholesterol: 60mg
- Sodium: 300mg
- Fiber: 3g
- Sugar: 15g

COCONUT-CRUSTED TILAPIA

Meal Description: Transport your taste buds to the tropics with Coconut-Crusted Tilapia—a delicious and crispy seafood dish that combines the mildness of tilapia with the sweetness of coconut. This recipe brings a tropical flair to your dinner table and is quick and easy to prepare.

Ingredients:

For the Coconut-Crusted Tilapia:

• Four tilapia fillets

• 1 cup shredded coconut (unsweetened)

• 1/2 cup breadcrumbs

• 1/4 cup all-purpose flour

• Two eggs, beaten

• One teaspoon of garlic powder

• One teaspoon of onion powder

• Salt and black pepper to taste

• Vegetable oil for frying

For the Mango Salsa:

• One ripe mango, peeled, pitted, and diced

- 1/2 red bell pepper, diced

- 1/4 cup red onion, finely chopped

- 1/4 cup fresh cilantro, chopped

- Juice of 1 lime

- Salt to taste

Instructions:

- Prepare the Mango Salsa:

- Combine diced mango, red bell pepper, red onion, cilantro, lime juice, and salt in a bowl. Mix well and refrigerate until ready to serve.

- Prepare the Coconut-Crusted Tilapia:

- In three separate shallow dishes, place flour in one, beaten eggs in another, and a mixture of shredded coconut, breadcrumbs, garlic powder, onion powder, salt, and black pepper in the third.

- Coat the Tilapia:

- Dip each tilapia fillet into the flour, shaking off excess.

- Dip the floured fillet into the beaten eggs, ensuring it is well-coated.

- Press the fillet into the coconut-breadcrumb mixture, covering it evenly on both sides.

- Fry the Tilapia:

- In a large skillet, heat vegetable oil over medium-high heat.

- Fry the coated tilapia fillets for 3-4 minutes per side or until they are golden brown and cooked through.

- Serve:

- Remove the coconut-crusted tilapia from the skillet and place them on a paper towel to absorb any excess oil.

- Serve the tilapia fillets with a side of mango salsa.

Nutrition Information (Per Serving):

- Calories: 350

- Protein: 25g

- Carbohydrates: 25g

- Fat: 18g

- Saturated Fat: 12g

- Cholesterol: 90mg

- Sodium: 300mg

- Fiber: 4g

- Sugar: 10g

GARLIC BUTTER SHRIMP STIR-FRY

Meal Description: Indulge in the rich and savory flavors of Garlic Butter Shrimp Stir-Fry—a quick and delicious dish that combines succulent shrimp with vibrant vegetables in a luscious garlic butter sauce. This recipe is perfect for a speedy weeknight dinner that doesn't compromise on taste.

Ingredients:

For the Garlic Butter Shrimp:

• 1 lb (450g) large shrimp, peeled and deveined

• Three tablespoons unsalted butter

• Four cloves garlic, minced

• One teaspoon of ginger, minced

• One tablespoon of soy sauce

• One tablespoon of oyster sauce

• One teaspoon of fish sauce (optional)

• One teaspoon cornstarch

• Salt and black pepper to taste

• Crushed red pepper flakes (optional for heat)

For the stir-fried vegetables:

- 2 cups broccoli florets

- One bell pepper, thinly sliced

- One carrot, julienned

- 1 cup snap peas, ends trimmed

- Two tablespoons of vegetable oil

For Garnish:

- Fresh cilantro, chopped

- Green onions, sliced

- Sesame seeds (optional)

For Serving:

- Cooked rice or noodles

Instructions:

- Prepare the Garlic Butter Shrimp:

- Mix shrimp with soy sauce, oyster sauce, fish sauce (if using), cornstarch, salt, and black pepper in a bowl. Set aside.

- In a large skillet or wok, melt butter over medium-high heat. Add minced garlic and ginger, sautéing until fragrant.

- Cook the Shrimp:

- Add the marinated shrimp to the skillet. Cook for 2-3 minutes on each side or until they turn pink and opaque. Remove the shrimp from the skillet and set aside.

- Stir-Fry Vegetables:

- In the same skillet, add vegetable oil. Stir-fry broccoli, bell pepper, carrot, and snap peas until they are crisp-tender but still vibrant in color.

• Combine Shrimp and Vegetables:

• Return the cooked shrimp to the skillet with the stir-fried vegetables. Toss to combine, ensuring everything is coated in the garlic butter sauce.

• Finish and Serve:

• Drizzle any remaining garlic butter sauce over the stir-fry. If desired, add crushed red pepper flakes for a touch of heat.

• Garnish with fresh cilantro, green onions, and sesame seeds.

• Serve Over Rice or Noodles:

• Serve the Garlic Butter Shrimp Stir-Fry over cooked rice or noodles.

Nutrition Information (Per Serving, excluding rice/ noodles):

• Calories: 300

• Protein: 25g

• Carbohydrates: 12g

• Fat: 18g

• Saturated Fat: 8g

• Cholesterol: 200mg

• Sodium: 700mg

• Fiber: 4g

• Sugar: 4g

BAKED COD WITH HERBED BREADCRUMBS

Meal Description: Savor the delicate flavor of Baked Cod with Herbed Breadcrumbs—a light and flaky fish dish that's elevated with a crispy herb-infused topping. This easy-to-make recipe is perfect for a wholesome, delicious, and nutritious dinner.

Ingredients:

For the Baked Cod:

• Four cod fillets (about 6 oz each)

• Two tablespoons of olive oil

• One tablespoon of lemon juice

• Salt and black pepper to taste

For the Herbed Breadcrumbs:

• 1 cup breadcrumbs (Panko or homemade)

• Two tablespoons fresh parsley, chopped

• One tablespoon of fresh dill, chopped

• One tablespoon of fresh chives chopped

• One teaspoon of lemon zest

• Two tablespoons melted butter

• Salt and black pepper to taste

For Serving:

• Lemon wedges

• Fresh herbs for garnish

Instructions:

• Preheat the Oven:

• Preheat your oven to 400°F (200°C).

• Prepare the Baked Cod:

• Pat the cod fillets dry with paper towels.

• Mix olive oil, lemon juice, salt, and black pepper in a small bowl.

• Brush the cod fillets with the olive oil mixture, ensuring they are evenly coated.

• Prepare the Herbed Breadcrumbs:

• Combine breadcrumbs, chopped parsley, chopped dill, chopped chives, lemon zest, melted butter, salt, and black pepper in another bowl. Mix well to create the herbed breadcrumbs mixture.

• Coat the Cod with Breadcrumbs:

• Press the herbed breadcrumbs mixture onto the top of each cod fillet, creating a generous coating.

• Bake in the Oven:

• Place the cod fillets on a baking sheet lined with parchment paper.

• Bake in the preheated oven for 12-15 minutes or until the fish is opaque and flakes easily with a fork.

- Serve:

- Remove the baked cod from the oven.

- Serve the cod fillets with lemon wedges and garnish with fresh herbs.

Nutrition Information (Per Serving):

- Calories: 250

- Protein: 30g

- Carbohydrates: 15g

- Fat: 9g

- Saturated Fat: 3g

- Cholesterol: 60mg

- Sodium: 400mg

- Fiber: 2g

- Sugar: 1g

SMOKED SALMON AND CREAM CHEESE BAGELS

Meal Description: Indulge in a classic and sophisticated brunch with Smoked Salmon and Cream Cheese Bagels. This iconic combination of rich smoked salmon and creamy cream cheese, paired with the chewiness of a bagel, creates a delightful symphony of flavors. Customize with your favorite toppings for a luxurious morning treat.

Ingredients:

• Four plain or everything bagels, sliced

• 8 oz (225g) smoked salmon

• 1 cup cream cheese, softened

• One red onion, thinly sliced

• One cucumber, thinly sliced

• Capers, for garnish

• Fresh dill for garnish

• Lemon wedges for serving

Instructions:

• Prepare the Bagels:

- Toast the bagel halves until golden brown.

- Spread Cream Cheese:

- Spread a generous layer of softened cream cheese on each bagel half.

- Assemble the Bagels:

- Arrange smoked salmon on top of the cream cheese-covered bagels.

- Add Toppings:

- Top the smoked salmon with thinly sliced red onions and cucumber.

- Garnish:

- Sprinkle capers over the bagels for a burst of salty flavor.

- Garnish with fresh dill for a touch of herbaceous goodness.

- Serve:

- Serve the Smoked Salmon and Cream Cheese Bagels with lemon wedges on the side.

Optional Additions:

- Sliced tomatoes

- Avocado slices

- Red pepper flakes for a hint of spice

- Freshly ground black pepper

Note: Feel free to customize the toppings based on your preferences. Whether you're enjoying a leisurely weekend brunch or a quick weekday treat, these Smoked Salmon and Cream Cheese Bagels are sure to elevate your morning.

Nutrition Information (Per Serving):

• Calories: 400

• Protein: 20g

• Carbohydrates: 40g

• Fat: 18g

• Saturated Fat: 8g

• Cholesterol: 50mg

• Sodium: 600mg

• Fiber: 3g

• Sugar: 2g

CHAPTER FIVE

Dairy Products Recipes

Greek Yogurt Parfait with Berries and Granola

Meal Description: Indulge in a wholesome and delightful Greek Yogurt Parfait with Berries and Granola— a nutritious and satisfying treat that's perfect for breakfast, a snack, or even a light dessert. Layered with creamy Greek yogurt, vibrant berries, and crunchy granola, this parfait is a burst of flavors and textures.

Ingredients:

• 2 cups Greek yogurt (unsweetened)

• 1 cup mixed berries (strawberries, blueberries, raspberries)

• 1/2 cup granola (homemade or store-bought)

• Two tablespoons honey or maple syrup (optional)

• Fresh mint leaves for garnish (optional)

Instructions:

• Prepare the Greek Yogurt:

• You may skip adding honey or maple syrup when using sweetened Greek yogurt. Otherwise, mix the honey or maple syrup into the unsweetened Greek yogurt for sweetness.

• Layer the Parfait:

• In serving glasses or bowls, begin by adding a layer of Greek yogurt at the bottom.

• Add Berries:

• Place a handful of mixed berries over the Greek yogurt layer.

- Sprinkle Granola:

- Add a layer of granola on top of the berries, creating a crunchy texture.

- Repeat Layers:

- Repeat the layers by adding more Greek yogurt, berries, and granola until you reach the top of the glass.

- Garnish and Drizzle (Optional):

- Garnish the top with a few additional berries and mint leaves for freshness.

- If desired, drizzle a bit of honey or maple syrup over the parfait.

- Serve:

- Serve the Greek Yogurt Parfait immediately for a delightful and nutritious treat.

Optional Additions:

- Chopped nuts (almonds, walnuts, or pecans)

- Shredded coconut

- Dried fruit (such as cranberries or raisins)

Note: Customize the parfait with your favorite toppings to suit your taste preferences. This Greek Yogurt Parfait with Berries and Granola is a versatile and satisfying option for any time of the day.

Nutrition Information (Per Serving):

- Calories: 300

- Protein: 15g

- Carbohydrates: 40g

- Fat: 10g

- Saturated Fat: 3g
- Cholesterol: 10mg
- Sodium: 50mg
- Fiber: 5g
- Sugar: 20g

COTTAGE CHEESE AND PINEAPPLE SMOOTHIE BOWL

Meal Description: Elevate your breakfast or snack with a refreshing, protein-packed Cottage Cheese and Pineapple Smoothie Bowl. This delightful bowl combines the creaminess of cottage cheese, the sweetness of pineapple, and the goodness of other nutritious ingredients for a satisfying and tropical treat.

Ingredients:

For the Smoothie Bowl:

• 1 cup cottage cheese

• 1 cup frozen pineapple chunks

• One ripe banana, sliced

• 1/2 cup almond milk (or any milk of your choice)

• One tablespoon of honey or maple syrup (optional for added sweetness)

• Ice cubes (optional)

For Toppings:

• Fresh pineapple chunks

• Sliced banana

• Granola

• Shredded coconut

• Chia seeds

• Mint leaves for garnish

Instructions:

• Prepare the Smoothie Base:

• In a blender, combine cottage cheese, frozen pineapple chunks, sliced banana, almond milk, and honey or maple syrup (if using).

• Blend until smooth and creamy. Add ice cubes if a thicker consistency is desired.

• Assemble the Smoothie Bowl:

• Pour the smoothie into a bowl.

• Add Toppings:

• Top the smoothie bowl with fresh pineapple chunks, sliced banana, granola, shredded coconut, chia seeds, and any other desired toppings.

• Garnish:

• Garnish with mint leaves for a burst of freshness.

• Serve:

• Serve the Cottage Cheese and Pineapple Smoothie Bowl immediately with a spoon.

Optional Additions:

• Nuts (such as almonds or walnuts)

• Berries (such as blueberries or strawberries)

• Drizzle of nut butter (peanut butter or almond butter)

• Edible flowers for decoration

Note: Feel free to customize the smoothie bowl with your favorite toppings and additions. This Cottage Cheese and Pineapple Smoothie Bowl is delicious and packed with protein and nutrients to kickstart your day.

Nutrition Information (Approximate):

• Calories: 350

• Protein: 20g

• Carbohydrates: 50g

• Fat: 8g

• Saturated Fat: 3g

• Cholesterol: 20mg

• Sodium: 400mg

• Fiber: 6g

• Sugar: 30g

SPINACH AND FETA STUFFED CHICKEN BREAST

Meal Description: Elevate your dinner with delicious, elegant spinach and feta-stuffed chicken breast. This recipe combines tender chicken breasts with a flavorful filling of spinach and feta, creating a savory and satisfying dish that's perfect for a special occasion or a delightful weeknight dinner.

Ingredients:

For the Stuffed Chicken:

- Four boneless, skinless chicken breasts

- 2 cups fresh spinach, chopped

- 1/2 cup crumbled feta cheese

- Two cloves garlic, minced

- One tablespoon of olive oil

- One teaspoon dried oregano

- Salt and black pepper to taste

For the Chicken Seasoning:

- One teaspoon paprika

- One teaspoon of garlic powder
- One teaspoon of onion powder
- Salt and black pepper to taste

For Pan Searing:

- Two tablespoons of olive oil

Instructions:

- Preheat the Oven:
- Preheat your oven to 375°F (190°C).
- Prepare the Spinach and Feta Filling:
- In a skillet, heat one tablespoon of olive oil over medium heat. Add minced garlic and sauté until fragrant.
- Add chopped spinach to the skillet and cook until wilted.
- Remove the skillet from heat and stir in crumbled feta, dried oregano, salt, and black pepper. Allow the mixture to cool.
- Prepare the Chicken Breasts:
- To create a pocket, butterfly each chicken breast by making a horizontal cut along the side without cutting all the way through.
- Stuff the Chicken:
- Stuff each chicken breast with the spinach and feta mixture, pressing the edges to seal.
- Season the Chicken:
- Mix paprika, garlic powder, onion powder, salt, and black pepper in a small bowl. Season both sides of each stuffed chicken breast with the spice mixture.
- Pan Sear the Chicken:

• Heat two tablespoons of olive oil over medium-high heat in an oven-safe skillet.

• Sear the stuffed chicken breasts for 2-3 minutes on each side until golden brown.

• Finish in the Oven:

• Transfer the skillet to the preheated oven and bake for 20-25 minutes or until the chicken is cooked through.

• Serve:

• Remove from the oven and let the chicken rest for a few minutes.

• Slice and serve the Spinach and Feta Stuffed Chicken Breast with your favorite side dishes.

Optional:

• Drizzle with a balsamic reduction or lemon butter sauce before serving.

• Garnish with fresh herbs, such as parsley or dill.

Note: Ensure the chicken reaches an internal temperature of 165°F (74°C) for safe consumption.

Nutrition Information (Per Serving):

• Calories: 300

• Protein: 35g

• Carbohydrates: 3g

• Fat: 16g

• Saturated Fat: 5g

• Cholesterol: 100mg

• Sodium: 400mg

• Fiber: 2g

- Sugar: 1g

CREAMY BROCCOLI AND CHEDDAR SOUP

Meal Description: Warm up with a comforting Creamy Broccoli and Cheddar Soup bowl. This classic soup combines the goodness of fresh broccoli with rich, melted cheddar cheese for a satisfying and flavorful experience. This homemade soup is sure to become a favorite for a cozy lunch or dinner.

Ingredients:

• Two tablespoons unsalted butter

• One onion, chopped

• Two cloves garlic, minced

• 3 cups fresh broccoli, chopped

• 3 cups low-sodium chicken or vegetable broth

• 1 cup milk (whole or 2%)

• 1/2 cup heavy cream (optional for extra creaminess)

• 2 cups sharp cheddar cheese, shredded

• 1/4 cup all-purpose flour

• Salt and black pepper to taste

• 1/4 teaspoon nutmeg (optional)

• Croutons or additional shredded cheddar for garnish (optional)

Instructions:

• Sauté Vegetables:

• In a large pot, melt the butter over medium heat. Add chopped onions and sauté until translucent. Add minced garlic and cook for an additional 1-2 minutes.

• Add Broccoli:

• Add chopped broccoli to the pot and cook for 5 minutes, stirring occasionally.

• Make Roux:

• Sprinkle flour over the vegetables and stir to coat evenly. Cook for 2-3 minutes to eliminate the raw flour taste.

• Add Liquid Ingredients:

• Gradually pour in the chicken or vegetable broth, stirring constantly to avoid lumps. Add milk and heavy cream (if using). Bring the mixture to a simmer.

• Simmer and Season:

• Let the soup simmer for 15-20 minutes or until the broccoli is tender. Season with salt, black pepper, and nutmeg (if using).

• Blend or Leave Chunky:

• For a smoother texture, use an immersion blender to puree the soup. Alternatively, leave the soup chunky for a heartier consistency.

• Add Cheddar Cheese:

• Reduce heat to low and gradually add shredded cheddar

cheese, stirring until melted and incorporated.

• Adjust Consistency:

• Add more broth or milk to reach your desired consistency if the soup is too thick.

• Serve:

• Ladle the Creamy Broccoli and Cheddar Soup into bowls. Garnish with croutons or additional shredded cheddar if desired.

Optional Additions:

• Crispy bacon bits

• Chopped green onions

• A dash of hot sauce for heat

Note: Adjust the seasoning and thickness according to your preference. This soup pairs well with crusty bread or a side salad for a complete meal.

Nutrition Information (Per Serving):

• Calories: 300

• Protein: 15g

• Carbohydrates: 20g

• Fat: 20g

• Saturated Fat: 12g

• Cholesterol: 60mg

• Sodium: 600mg

• Fiber: 4g

• Sugar: 6g

CHEESY BAKED ZITI WITH RICOTTA

Meal Description: Indulge in comfort food with Cheesy Baked Ziti with Ricotta. This classic Italian-American dish brings together perfectly cooked ziti pasta, a rich tomato sauce, a blend of melted cheeses, and creamy ricotta for a hearty and satisfying meal. Gather the family for a delightful dinner that will become a favorite.

Ingredients:

For the Baked Ziti:

• 1 pound (450g) ziti pasta

• One tablespoon of olive oil

• One onion, finely chopped

• Three cloves garlic, minced

• 1 pound (450g) ground beef or Italian sausage (optional)

• One can (28 ounces) crushed tomatoes

• One can (15 ounces) of tomato sauce

• One teaspoon dried oregano

• One teaspoon of dried basil

• Salt and black pepper to taste

For the Cheesy Layer:

• 2 cups shredded mozzarella cheese

• 1 cup grated Parmesan cheese

For the Ricotta Mixture:

• 2 cups ricotta cheese

• One egg

• 1/4 cup fresh parsley, chopped

• Salt and black pepper to taste

Instructions:

• Preheat the Oven:

• Preheat your oven to 375°F (190°C).

• Cook Ziti:

• Cook the ziti pasta according to the package instructions. Drain and set aside.

• Prepare the Sauce:

• In a large skillet, heat olive oil over medium heat. Add chopped onion and sauté until translucent. Add minced garlic and cook for an additional minute.

• If using ground beef or sausage, add it to the skillet and cook until browned. Drain excess fat if necessary.

• Pour in crushed tomatoes and tomato sauce. Season with oregano, basil, salt, and black pepper. Simmer for 15-20 minutes.

• Make Ricotta Mixture:

• Combine ricotta cheese, egg, chopped parsley, salt, and black pepper in a bowl. Mix well.

• Assemble the Baked Ziti:

• Combine the cooked ziti with the tomato sauce mixture

in a large mixing bowl. Stir until the pasta is evenly coated.

• Layering:

• In a greased baking dish, spread half of the ziti mixture.

• Dollop half of the ricotta mixture on top and spread it evenly.

• Sprinkle half of the shredded mozzarella and grated Parmesan over the ricotta layer.

• Repeat the layers with the remaining ziti, ricotta, and cheese.

• Bake:

• Bake in the preheated oven for 25-30 minutes or until the cheese is melted and bubbly and the edges are golden.

• Serve:

• Allow the Cheesy Baked Ziti to cool for a few minutes before serving. Garnish with fresh parsley if desired.

Optional Additions:

• Sautéed mushrooms or bell peppers

• Crushed red pepper flakes for a touch of heat

Note: Customize the recipe by adding your favorite ingredients to the sauce or adjusting the level of spiciness.

Nutrition Information (Per Serving):

• Calories: 450

• Protein: 25g

• Carbohydrates: 40g

• Fat: 20g

- Saturated Fat: 10g
- Cholesterol: 90mg
- Sodium: 800mg
- Fiber: 4g
- Sugar: 8g

YOGURT-MARINATED CHICKEN SKEWERS

Meal Description: Treat your taste buds to the delightful flavors of Yogurt-Marinated Chicken Skewers. This recipe features tender chicken pieces marinated in a rich and aromatic yogurt blend, resulting in juicy, flavorful skewers that are perfect for grilling or baking. Whether served as a main dish or party appetizer, these skewers are sure to be a hit.

Ingredients:

For the Marinade:

• 1 cup plain Greek yogurt

• Two tablespoons of olive oil

• Three cloves garlic, minced

• One teaspoon of ground cumin

• One teaspoon of ground coriander

• One teaspoon of smoked paprika

• One teaspoon turmeric

• One teaspoon of ground black pepper

• One teaspoon salt

• Juice of 1 lemon

• Two tablespoons fresh cilantro, chopped (optional)

For the Chicken:

• 1.5 lbs (700g) boneless, skinless chicken breasts cut into bite-sized cubes

• Wooden or metal skewers, soaked in water if wooden

Instructions:

• Prepare the Marinade:

• In a bowl, combine Greek yogurt, olive oil, minced garlic, cumin, coriander, smoked paprika, turmeric, black pepper, salt, lemon juice, and chopped cilantro (if using). Mix well to create a smooth marinade.

• Marinate the Chicken:

• Place the chicken cubes in the marinade, ensuring they are well-coated. Cover the bowl with plastic wrap and refrigerate for at least 1-2 hours or overnight for maximum flavor.

• Skewer the Chicken:

• Preheat your grill or oven to medium-high heat.

• Thread the marinated chicken cubes onto the skewers, leaving a little space between each piece.

• Grill or Bake:

• If grilling, cook the skewers for 10-15 minutes, turning occasionally, until the chicken is cooked through and has a nice char.

• If baking, place the skewers on a lined baking sheet and bake in a preheated oven at 400°F (200°C) for 20-25 minutes or until the chicken is cooked through.

• Serve:

• Once cooked, remove the Yogurt-Marinated Chicken Skewers from the grill or oven.

• Serve hot with your favorite side dishes, such as rice, salad, or a yogurt sauce.

Optional Additions:

• Serve with a side of tzatziki sauce or yogurt-based dip.

• Garnish with extra fresh cilantro or a squeeze of lemon juice before serving.

Note: These Yogurt-Marinated Chicken Skewers are versatile and can be enjoyed on their own or paired with a variety of sides for a complete and satisfying meal.

Nutrition Information (Per Serving):

• Calories: 250

• Protein: 30g

• Carbohydrates: 5g

• Fat: 12g

• Saturated Fat: 2.5g

• Cholesterol: 80mg

• Sodium: 500mg

• Fiber: 1g

• Sugar: 2g

CHILLED CUCUMBER AND YOGURT SOUP

Meal Description: Cool down with the refreshing taste of Chilled Cucumber and Yogurt Soup. This light and creamy soup, infused with the crispness of cucumbers and the tanginess of yogurt, is a perfect dish for warm days. Serve it as a refreshing appetizer or enjoy it as a light lunch—either way, it's a delightful culinary experience.

Ingredients:

- Two large cucumbers, peeled and diced

- 2 cups plain Greek yogurt

- 1 cup cold water

- Two tablespoons fresh mint, chopped

- One clove of garlic, minced

- One tablespoon of olive oil

- One tablespoon of fresh lemon juice

- Salt and black pepper to taste

- Optional Garnish: Additional chopped cucumber, mint leaves, and a drizzle of olive oil

Instructions:

- Prepare Cucumbers:

- Peel and dice the cucumbers. Reserve a small portion for garnish if desired.

- Blend Ingredients:

- Combine the diced cucumbers, Greek yogurt, cold water, chopped mint, minced garlic, olive oil, and fresh lemon juice in a blender.

- Blend Until Smooth:

- Blend the ingredients until smooth and creamy. If the soup is too thick, you can add more cold water until the desired consistency is reached.

- Season:

- Season the soup with salt and black pepper. Adjust the seasoning according to your taste preferences.

- Chill:

- Transfer the soup to a bowl and refrigerate for at least 2 hours or until well-chilled.

- Serve:

- Before serving, give the soup a good stir. Ladle the Chilled Cucumber and Yogurt Soup into bowls.

- Garnish (Optional):

- Garnish each serving with additional diced cucumber, mint leaves, and a drizzle of olive oil.

- Enjoy:

- Serve the Chilled Cucumber and Yogurt Soup as a refreshing appetizer or light lunch.

Optional Additions:

• A pinch of cayenne pepper or chili flakes for a hint of heat.

• Diced avocado for extra creaminess.

• Croutons or a swirl of balsamic glaze for added texture and flavor.

Note: This soup is best served cold, making it a perfect choice for hot summer days. Customize the garnishes and seasonings to suit your taste preferences.

Nutrition Information (Per Serving):

• Calories: 120

• Protein: 10g

• Carbohydrates: 10g

• Fat: 5g

• Saturated Fat: 1g

• Cholesterol: 5mg

• Sodium: 50mg

• Fiber: 2g

• Sugar: 6g

CREAMY MUSHROOM AND SWISS CHICKEN

Meal Description: Indulge in a comforting and elegant dish with Creamy Mushroom and Swiss Chicken. This recipe features tender chicken breasts smothered in rich, velvety mushroom and Swiss cheese sauce. Serve it over pasta, rice, or a side of vegetables for a delicious and satisfying dinner.

Ingredients:

For the Chicken:

- Four boneless, skinless chicken breasts

- Salt and black pepper to taste

- One teaspoon of garlic powder

- One teaspoon paprika

- Two tablespoons of olive oil

For the Creamy Mushroom and Swiss Sauce:

- Two tablespoons butter

- 8 oz (225g) cremini or white mushrooms, sliced

- Three cloves garlic, minced

- 1 cup chicken broth

- 1 cup heavy cream

- 1 cup Swiss cheese, shredded

- Salt and black pepper to taste

- Fresh parsley, chopped, for garnish

Instructions:

- Season and Sear the Chicken:

- Season chicken breasts with salt, black pepper, garlic powder, and paprika.

- In a large skillet, heat olive oil over medium-high heat. Sear the chicken breasts for 4-5 minutes on each side or until golden brown and cooked through. Remove from the skillet and set aside.

- Make the Mushroom Sauce:

- In the same skillet, add butter. Once melted, add sliced mushrooms and sauté until they release their moisture and become golden brown.

- Add minced garlic and sauté for an additional 1-2 minutes until fragrant.

- Deglaze with Broth:

- Pour in chicken broth, scraping the bottom of the skillet to release any browned bits. Allow it to simmer for 2-3 minutes.

- Add Cream and Cheese:

- Lower the heat and pour in heavy cream. Stir in shredded Swiss cheese until it melts and the sauce becomes creamy.

- Season and Simmer:

• Season the sauce with salt and black pepper to taste. Simmer for 2-3 minutes until the sauce thickens.

• Combine Chicken and Sauce:

• Return the seared chicken breasts to the skillet, coating them with the creamy mushroom and Swiss sauce. Let it simmer for an additional 5 minutes to allow the flavors to meld.

• Garnish and Serve:

• Garnish with chopped fresh parsley and serve the Creamy Mushroom and Swiss Chicken over pasta, rice, or with your favorite side dishes.

Optional Additions:

• Sautéed spinach or asparagus for added greens.

• A splash of white wine for extra depth of flavor.

Note: Adjust the thickness of the sauce by adding more or less chicken broth and heavy cream. Customize the seasoning to your taste.

Nutrition Information (Per Serving):

• Calories: 450

• Protein: 30g

• Carbohydrates: 5g

• Fat: 35g

• Saturated Fat: 18g

• Cholesterol: 150mg

• Sodium: 600mg

• Fiber: 1g

• Sugar: 2g

CHAPTER SIX

Eggs Recipes

Spinach and Mushroom Omelette

Meal Description: Start your day with a nutritious and flavorful Spinach and Mushroom Omelette. This quick and easy breakfast recipe combines the earthy goodness of mushrooms with the leafy greens of spinach, all enveloped in a fluffy omelet. Packed with protein and vitamins, this omelet is a delicious way to kickstart your morning.

Ingredients:

• Three large eggs

• Salt and black pepper to taste

• One tablespoon of butter or olive oil

• 1/2 cup mushrooms, sliced

• 1 cup fresh spinach, chopped

• 1/4 cup feta cheese, crumbled (optional)

• One tablespoon of fresh chives chopped (for garnish, optional)

• Salsa or hot sauce (optional for serving)

Instructions:

• Prepare the Eggs:

• Crack the eggs into a bowl, season with salt and black pepper, and whisk until well beaten.

• Sauté Mushrooms and Spinach:

• In a non-stick skillet, heat butter or olive oil over medium heat. Add sliced mushrooms and cook until they release their moisture and become golden brown.

• Add chopped spinach to the skillet and sauté until wilted. Remove mushrooms and spinach from the skillet and set aside.

• Cook the Omelette:

• Add more butter or oil, if needed, in the same skillet. Pour the beaten eggs into the skillet, tilting it to spread the eggs evenly.

• Add Filling:

• Once the edges of the omelet start to set, spoon the sautéed mushrooms and spinach onto one half of the omelet.

• Add Cheese (Optional):

• Sprinkle crumbled feta cheese over the mushroom and spinach mixture.

• Fold and Cook:

• Gently fold the other half of the omelet over the filling, creating a half-moon shape. Allow it to cook for an additional 1-2 minutes until the eggs are fully set.

• Garnish and Serve:

• Slide the omelet onto a plate. Garnish with fresh chives if desired. Serve hot with salsa or hot sauce on the side if you like a bit of heat.

Optional Additions:

• Diced tomatoes or cherry tomatoes for a burst of freshness.

• A sprinkle of shredded cheddar or mozzarella cheese for added meltiness.

• Sautéed onions or bell peppers for extra flavor.

Note: Customize the omelet with your favorite ingredients and seasonings.

Nutrition Information (Approximate):

• Calories: 300

• Protein: 18g

• Carbohydrates: 5g

• Fat: 24g

• Saturated Fat: 10g

• Cholesterol: 470mg

• Sodium: 400mg

• Fiber: 2g

• Sugar: 2g

EGG SALAD SANDWICHES

Meal Description: Savor the classic and satisfying flavor of Egg Salad Sandwiches. This simple recipe transforms hard-boiled eggs into a creamy and delicious filling, perfect for a quick and wholesome lunch. Spread it between slices of your favorite bread, and you've got a timeless, comforting, nutritious, timeless sandwich.

Ingredients:

For the Egg Salad:

• Six hard-boiled eggs, peeled and chopped

• 1/4 cup mayonnaise

• One tablespoon of Dijon mustard

• 1/4 cup celery, finely diced

• Two tablespoons red onion, finely chopped

• One tablespoon of fresh dill, chopped

• Salt and black pepper to taste

For the Sandwiches:

• Sliced bread (white, whole wheat, or your preference)

• Lettuce leaves

• Tomato slices

• Additional mayonnaise or mustard for spreading (optional)

Instructions:

• Prepare the Egg Salad:

• Combine chopped hard-boiled eggs, mayonnaise, Dijon mustard, diced celery, chopped red onion, and fresh dill in a mixing bowl.

• Mix the ingredients until well combined. Season with salt and black pepper to taste. Adjust mayonnaise and mustard quantities based on your desired creaminess and tanginess.

• Assemble the Sandwiches:

• Spread a generous portion of the egg salad onto one slice of bread.

• Add Fresh Ingredients:

• Layer with lettuce leaves and tomato slices for added freshness and crunch.

• Top and Serve:

• Place another slice of bread on top to create a sandwich. Press gently.

• Optional Spreads:

• If desired, spread additional mayonnaise or mustard on the second slice of bread for extra flavor.

• Slice and Enjoy:

• Using a sharp knife, slice the Egg Salad Sandwich in half diagonally or straight across. Serve immediately.

Optional Additions:

• A dash of hot sauce or a sprinkle of paprika for a hint of spice.

• Sliced avocado or cucumber for added creaminess or crunch.

• Pickles or relish for a tangy twist.

Note: Customize the egg salad with your preferred herbs and spices. Enjoy this classic Egg Salad Sandwich as a quick and delicious meal.

Nutrition Information (Approximate per Sandwich):

• Calories: 350

• Protein: 15g

• Carbohydrates: 25g

• Fat: 20g

• Saturated Fat: 4g

• Cholesterol: 370mg

• Sodium: 600mg

• Fiber: 3g

• Sugar: 4g

SHAKSHUKA (POACHED EGGS IN SPICY TOMATO SAUCE)

Meal Description: Transport your taste buds to the Mediterranean with Shakshuka, a flavorful dish featuring poached eggs in spicy and aromatic tomato sauce. Bursting with vibrant colors and rich flavors, Shakshuka is perfect for brunch or a hearty breakfast. Serve it with crusty bread to soak up the savory sauce.

Ingredients:

- Two tablespoons of olive oil
- One onion, finely chopped
- One red bell pepper, diced
- Two cloves garlic, minced
- One teaspoon of ground cumin
- One teaspoon of smoked paprika
- 1/2 teaspoon chili powder (adjust to taste)
- One can (28 ounces) crushed tomatoes
- Salt and black pepper to taste

- 4-6 large eggs

- Fresh parsley, chopped, for garnish

- Feta cheese, crumbled (optional, for garnish)

- Crusty bread or pita for serving

Instructions:

- Sauté Vegetables:

- Heat olive oil over medium heat in a large skillet or cast-iron pan. Add finely chopped onion and diced red bell pepper. Sauté until the vegetables are softened, about 5 minutes.

- Add Aromatics and Spices:

- Add minced garlic, ground cumin, smoked paprika, and chili powder to the skillet. Stir and cook for an additional 1-2 minutes until fragrant.

- Tomato Sauce:

- Pour in the crushed tomatoes and season with salt and black pepper. Simmer the sauce for 10-15 minutes until it thickens.

- Create Wells for Eggs:

- Make small wells in the tomato sauce for each egg using a spoon. Crack the eggs into the wells.

- Poach the Eggs:

- Cover the skillet with a lid and let the eggs poach in the simmering tomato sauce for 5-7 minutes or until the egg whites are set but the yolks are still runny.

- Garnish and Serve:

- Garnish the Shakshuka with chopped fresh parsley and crumbled feta cheese (if using). Serve hot with crusty bread or pita on the side.

Optional Additions:

• Sliced olives or capers for a salty kick.

• Chopped fresh cilantro or mint for additional freshness.

• A sprinkle of red pepper flakes for extra heat.

Note: Adjust the spice level according to your preference. Shakshuka can be made milder or spicier based on the amount of chili powder used.

Nutrition Information (Approximate per Serving):

• Calories: 250

• Protein: 12g

• Carbohydrates: 15g

• Fat: 15g

• Saturated Fat: 3g

• Cholesterol: 190mg

• Sodium: 700mg

• Fiber: 4g

• Sugar: 8g

ASPARAGUS AND FETA FRITTATA

Meal Description: Elevate your breakfast or brunch with the delightful combination of Asparagus and Feta Frittata. This easy-to-make dish features tender asparagus spears and creamy feta cheese baked into a fluffy and flavorful frittata. Serve it as a main course or slice it into wedges for a delightful addition to a brunch spread.

Ingredients:

• One bunch of asparagus, trimmed and cut into bite-sized pieces

• Eight large eggs

• 1/4 cup milk

• Salt and black pepper to taste

• One tablespoon of olive oil

• One small onion, finely chopped

• Two cloves garlic, minced

• 1/2 cup feta cheese, crumbled

• Fresh parsley, chopped, for garnish (optional)

Instructions:

• Preheat Oven:

- Preheat your oven to 375°F (190°C).

- Blanch Asparagus:

- Bring a pot of salted water to a boil. Add the asparagus pieces and blanch for 2-3 minutes until they are bright green and slightly tender. Drain and set aside.

- Whisk Eggs:

- Whisk together eggs, milk, salt, and black pepper in a bowl until well combined. Set aside.

- Sauté Vegetables:

- In an oven-safe skillet, heat olive oil over medium heat. Add finely chopped onion and sauté until softened, about 3 minutes. Add minced garlic and cook for an additional 1-2 minutes.

- Add Asparagus:

- Add the blanched asparagus pieces to the skillet and sauté for another 2 minutes.

- Pour Egg Mixture:

- Pour the whisked egg mixture over the vegetables in the skillet. Allow it to set for a minute, gently lifting the edges with a spatula to let the uncooked eggs flow underneath.

- Add Feta Cheese:

- Sprinkle crumbled feta cheese evenly over the top of the frittata.

- Bake:

- Transfer the skillet to the preheated oven and bake for 15-20 minutes or until the frittata is set in the middle and the edges are golden brown.

- Garnish and Serve:

• Remove from the oven and let it cool slightly. Garnish with fresh parsley if desired. Cut into wedges and serve warm.

Optional Additions:

• Cherry tomatoes or sun-dried tomatoes for added sweetness.

• Sautéed mushrooms for an earthy flavor.

• Fresh dill or thyme for additional herbaceous notes.

Note: Customize the frittata with your favorite vegetables and herbs.

Nutrition Information (Approximate per Serving):

• Calories: 200

• Protein: 15g

• Carbohydrates: 5g

• Fat: 14g

• Saturated Fat: 5g

• Cholesterol: 330mg

• Sodium: 350mg

• Fiber: 2g

• Sugar: 2g

HUEVOS RANCHEROS

Meal Description: Experience Mexico's bold and vibrant flavors with Huevos Rancheros, a classic breakfast dish featuring fried eggs served on a bed of warm tortillas, smothered in a rich tomato-chili sauce. This hearty and flavorful meal is often garnished with beans, avocado, and cheese, creating a satisfying and delicious start to your day.

Ingredients:

- Four corn tortillas

- Four large eggs

- One tablespoon of vegetable oil

- One onion, finely chopped

- Two cloves garlic, minced

- One can (14 ounces) crushed tomatoes

- One teaspoon of ground cumin

- One teaspoon of chili powder

- Salt and black pepper to taste

- One can (15 ounces) black beans, drained and rinsed

- One avocado, sliced

• Fresh cilantro, chopped, for garnish

• Queso fresco or shredded cheese for garnish (optional)

• Lime wedges for serving

Instructions:

• Prepare Tortillas:

• Heat the corn tortillas in a dry skillet or over an open flame until warm and slightly toasted. Keep them warm by wrapping them in a kitchen towel.

• Fry Eggs:

• In the same skillet, heat vegetable oil over medium heat. Fry the eggs to your desired doneness, keeping the yolks runny for the traditional style.

• Sauté Onion and Garlic:

• In a separate saucepan, sauté finely chopped onion in a bit of oil until softened. Add minced garlic and cook for another minute.

• Make Tomato-Chili Sauce:

• Pour the crushed tomatoes and season with ground cumin, chili powder, salt, and black pepper. Simmer the sauce for 10-15 minutes until it thickens.

• Warm Black Beans:

• Heat the black beans over low heat in a small saucepan until warmed through.

• Assemble Huevos Rancheros:

• Place a warm tortilla on each plate. Spoon a generous portion of the tomato-chili sauce over the tortilla.

• Top with a fried egg, and add a scoop of black beans on the side.

• Garnish:

• Garnish with sliced avocado, chopped cilantro, and queso fresco or shredded cheese if desired.

• Serve:

• Serve the Huevos Rancheros immediately, accompanied by lime wedges for squeezing over the dish.

Optional Additions:

• Salsa or pico de gallo for added freshness and spice.

• Jalapeño slices for extra heat.

• Guacamole for a creamy and flavorful topping.

Note: Customize the dish based on your preferences for spiciness and toppings.

Nutrition Information (Approximate per Serving):

• Calories: 400

• Protein: 16g

• Carbohydrates: 40g

• Fat: 20g

• Saturated Fat: 4g

• Cholesterol: 195mg

• Sodium: 700mg

• Fiber: 12g

• Sugar: 5g

DEVILED EGGS WITH SMOKED PAPRIKA

Appetizer Description: Elevate a classic appetizer with these Deviled Eggs featuring a hint of smokiness from smoked paprika. Creamy, tangy, and beautifully seasoned, these deviled eggs are a crowd-pleaser at any gathering or party. They make a delightful addition to your appetizer spread and are sure to disappear quickly.

Ingredients:

• Six hard-boiled eggs peeled

• 1/4 cup mayonnaise

• One teaspoon of Dijon mustard

• One teaspoon of white vinegar

• Salt and black pepper to taste

• 1/2 teaspoon smoked paprika, plus extra for garnish

• Fresh chives or parsley, chopped, for garnish

Instructions:

• Prepare Hard-Boiled Eggs:

• Boil eggs until hard-cooked, approximately 10-12 minutes. Once cooked, cool, peel, and cut them in half lengthwise.

• Remove Yolks:

• Carefully remove the egg yolks and place them in a bowl.

• Make Filling:

• Mash the egg yolks with a fork. Add mayonnaise, Dijon mustard, white vinegar, salt, black pepper, and smoked paprika to the mashed yolks. Mix until well combined and smooth.

• Fill Egg Whites:

• Spoon or pipe the yolk mixture back into the egg white halves. You can use a piping or zip-top bag with the corner snipped off for a neater presentation.

• Garnish:

• Sprinkle the deviled eggs with additional smoked paprika for a smoky finish. Garnish with chopped fresh chives or parsley.

• Chill and Serve:

• Refrigerate the deviled eggs for at least 30 minutes before serving to allow the flavors to meld and the filling to set.

• Serve:

• Arrange the Deviled Eggs on a serving platter and serve chilled.

Optional Additions:

• Finely chopped pickles or relish for a tangy twist.

• A dash of hot sauce for a spicy kick.

• Crumbled bacon for added richness and flavor.

Note: Adjust the seasoning and filling consistency to your taste.

Nutrition Information (Approximate, per Serving - 2 halves):

- Calories: 120

- Protein: 6g

- Carbohydrates: 1g

- Fat: 10g

- Saturated Fat: 2g

- Cholesterol: 190mg

- Sodium: 110mg

- Fiber: 0g

- Sugar: 0g

VEGGIE AND CHEESE STUFFED BREAKFAST BURRITOS

Meal Description: Kickstart your day with a satisfying and flavorful breakfast by indulging in these Veggie and Cheese Stuffed Breakfast Burritos. Packed with a medley of colorful vegetables, scrambled eggs, and melted cheese, these burritos are a delicious and portable morning treat. Customize the fillings to suit your taste, and enjoy a hearty and nutritious breakfast on the go.

Ingredients:

• Four large flour tortillas

• Six large eggs, beaten

• One tablespoon of olive oil

• One bell pepper, diced (any color)

• One small red onion, finely chopped

• 1 cup cherry tomatoes, halved

• 1 cup baby spinach, chopped

• 1 cup shredded cheddar or Monterey Jack cheese

• Salt and black pepper to taste

• Salsa, guacamole, or sour cream for serving (optional)

Instructions:

• Sauté Vegetables:

• In a large skillet, heat olive oil over medium heat. Add diced bell pepper and chopped red onion. Sauté until the vegetables are softened, about 3-5 minutes.

• Add Tomatoes and Spinach:

• Add halved cherry tomatoes to the skillet and cook for 2 minutes until they soften. Stir in chopped baby spinach and cook until wilted.

• Scramble Eggs:

• Push the sautéed vegetables to one side of the skillet and pour the beaten eggs into the empty side. Scramble the eggs until cooked through, combining them with the vegetables.

• Season and Melt Cheese:

• Season the egg and vegetable mixture with salt and black pepper to taste. Sprinkle shredded cheese over the top and let it melt, stirring to combine.

• Assemble Burritos:

• Warm the flour tortillas in a dry skillet or microwave. Place a portion of the egg and vegetable mixture in the center of each tortilla.

• Fold and Roll:

• Fold the sides of the tortilla inward and then roll it up from the bottom to create a burrito.

• Serve:

• Place the Veggie and Cheese Stuffed Breakfast Burritos seam-side down on a serving plate. Serve with salsa, guacamole, or sour cream on the side if desired.

Optional Additions:

• Black beans or refried beans for added protein.

• Sliced avocado or guacamole for creaminess.

• Sautéed mushrooms or zucchini for extra veggies.

Note: Customize the burritos with your favorite breakfast ingredients.

Nutrition Information (Approximate, per Burrito):

• Calories: 350

• Protein: 15g

• Carbohydrates: 25g

• Fat: 20g

• Saturated Fat: 8g

• Cholesterol: 280mg

• Sodium: 500mg

• Fiber: 3g

• Sugar: 3g

CLASSIC EGGS BENEDICT

Meal Description: Elevate your brunch experience with the timeless and indulgent Classic Eggs Benedict. This iconic dish features perfectly poached eggs nestled atop Canadian bacon and English muffins, all smothered in velvety hollandaise sauce. Impress your guests or treat yourself to this luxurious breakfast combining rich flavors and textures.

Ingredients:

For Eggs Benedict:

• Four large eggs

• 4 English muffins, split and toasted

• Eight slices of Canadian bacon or ham

• Fresh chives or parsley, chopped (for garnish)

• Salt and black pepper to taste

For Hollandaise Sauce:

• Three large egg yolks

• One tablespoon water

• One tablespoon of lemon juice

• 1 cup unsalted butter, melted

- Salt and cayenne pepper to taste

Instructions:

- Prepare Hollandaise Sauce:

- In a blender, combine egg yolks, water, and lemon juice. Blend until smooth.

- With the blender running, slowly stream in the melted butter until the sauce thickens. Season with salt and a pinch of cayenne pepper. Keep the hollandaise warm.

- Poach Eggs:

- Fill a wide, shallow pan with water and bring it to a gentle simmer. Add a splash of vinegar to help the eggs coagulate.

- Crack each egg into a small bowl. Create a gentle whirlpool in the simmering water and slide the egg into the center. Poach each egg for about 3-4 minutes for a runny yolk.

- Cook Canadian Bacon:

- While poaching eggs, heat a skillet and cook the Canadian bacon slices until warmed through and slightly browned.

- Assemble Eggs Benedict:

- Place toasted English muffin halves on a plate. Top each half with a slice of Canadian bacon.

- Carefully place a poached egg on top of each bacon-covered muffin half.

- Pour Hollandaise Sauce:

- Generously pour hollandaise sauce over each poached egg.

• Garnish and Serve:

• Garnish with chopped fresh chives or parsley. Season with salt and black pepper to taste. Serve immediately.

Optional Additions:

• Sautéed spinach or asparagus for added freshness.

• Smoked salmon or lox for a luxurious twist.

• A sprinkle of paprika or smoked paprika for extra flavor.

Note: Adjust the thickness of the hollandaise sauce by adding more or less melted butter.

Nutrition Information (Approximate per Serving):

• Calories: 500

• Protein: 15g

• Carbohydrates: 30g

• Fat: 35g

• Saturated Fat: 20g

• Cholesterol: 375mg

• Sodium: 700mg

• Fiber: 2g

• Sugar: 1g

CHAPTER SEVEN

Fortified Foods Recipes

Fortified Cereal Parfait with Almond Milk

Meal Description: Start your day with a nutritious and energizing Fortified Cereal Parfait with Almond Milk. This delightful parfait combines the goodness of fortified cereal, almond milk, and a medley of fresh fruits and nuts. It's a wholesome and satisfying breakfast that provides essential nutrients to kickstart your morning on a healthy note.

Ingredients:

• 1 cup fortified whole-grain cereal (such as bran flakes or whole-grain flakes)

• 1 cup unsweetened almond milk

• 1/2 cup Greek yogurt (optional)

• One tablespoon of chia seeds

• One tablespoon of honey or maple syrup (optional for sweetness)

• Fresh berries (strawberries, blueberries, raspberries)

• Sliced banana

• Two tablespoons chopped nuts (almonds, walnuts, or your choice)

• Fresh mint leaves for garnish (optional)

Instructions:

• Prepare the Cereal Base:

• In a bowl, combine fortified whole-grain cereal with almond milk. Let it soak for a few minutes to allow the cereal to absorb the almond milk.

- Add Chia Seeds:

- Stir in chia seeds and let the mixture sit for an additional 5 minutes. This allows the chia seeds to expand and add a delightful texture to the parfait.

- Layer with Greek Yogurt (Optional):

- If using Greek yogurt, layer a portion at the bottom of a glass or bowl.

- Alternate Layers:

- Start layering the cereal mixture, fresh berries, sliced banana, and chopped nuts in the glass or bowl. Repeat the layers until you reach the top.

- Drizzle with Honey or Maple Syrup (Optional):

- Drizzle honey or maple syrup over the top for added sweetness if desired.

- Garnish and Serve:

- Garnish the parfait with fresh mint leaves if desired. Serve immediately and enjoy a nutrient-packed breakfast.

Optional Additions:

- Unsweetened coconut flakes for a tropical twist.

- Diced mango or pineapple for added sweetness and flavor.

- A sprinkle of cinnamon or nutmeg for warm and cozy notes.

Note: Customize the parfait with your favorite fruits and toppings.

Nutrition Information (Approximate per Serving):

- Calories: 400

- Protein: 12g
- Carbohydrates: 60g
- Fat: 15g
- Saturated Fat: 1g
- Cholesterol: 0mg
- Sodium: 300mg
- Fiber: 10g
- Sugar: 15g

TOFU AND VEGETABLE STIR-FRY

Meal Description: Enjoy a delicious and wholesome Tofu and Vegetable Stir-Fry that's packed with protein and vibrant flavors. This quick and easy stir-fry combines tofu, colorful vegetables, and a savory stir-fry sauce for a satisfying and nutritious meal. Serve it over rice or noodles for a complete and hearty dinner.

Ingredients:

For the Stir-Fry:

• One block (14 ounces) of extra-firm tofu, pressed and cubed

• Two tablespoons of soy sauce

• One tablespoon cornstarch

• Two tablespoons vegetable oil divided

• One bell pepper, thinly sliced (any color)

• One carrot, julienned

• 1 cup broccoli florets

• 1 cup snap peas, ends trimmed

• Two cloves garlic, minced

• One tablespoon of fresh ginger, grated

• Sesame seeds and sliced green onions for garnish (optional)

For the Stir-Fry Sauce:

• Three tablespoons soy sauce

• Two tablespoons of hoisin sauce

• One tablespoon of rice vinegar

• One tablespoon of sesame oil

• One tablespoon of maple syrup or honey

• 1 teaspoon cornstarch

Instructions:

• Press Tofu:

• Press the tofu to remove excess water by wrapping it in a clean kitchen towel and placing a heavy object on top. Let it press for at least 15-20 minutes.

• Marinate Tofu:

• Mix cubed tofu with soy sauce and cornstarch in a bowl, ensuring the tofu is well coated. Let it marinate for 10-15 minutes.

• Prepare Stir-Fry Sauce:

• Whisk together soy sauce, hoisin sauce, rice vinegar, sesame oil, maple syrup (or honey), and cornstarch in a small bowl. Set aside.

• Sauté Tofu:

• Heat one tablespoon of vegetable oil in a large skillet or wok over medium-high heat. Add the marinated tofu and cook until golden brown on all sides. Remove tofu from the pan and set aside.

• Sauté Vegetables:

• In the same pan, add another tablespoon of oil. Sauté sliced bell pepper, julienned carrot, broccoli florets, and snap peas until they are tender-crisp.

• Add Aromatics:

• Stir in minced garlic and grated ginger, cooking for an additional minute until fragrant.

• Combine Tofu and Sauce:

• Add the cooked tofu back to the pan and pour the prepared stir-fry sauce over the tofu and vegetables. Toss everything together until well coated and heated through.

• Garnish and Serve:

• Garnish the Tofu and Vegetable Stir-Fry with sesame seeds and sliced green onions if desired. Serve over rice or noodles.

Optional Additions:

• Sliced mushrooms or baby corn for additional veggies.

• Cashews or peanuts for added crunch.

• Red pepper flakes for extra heat.

Note: Adjust the thickness of the sauce according to your preference by adding more or less cornstarch.

Nutrition Information (Approximate per Serving):

• Calories: 350

• Protein: 18g

• Carbohydrates: 25g

- Fat: 20g
- Saturated Fat: 2g
- Cholesterol: 0mg
- Sodium: 800mg
- Fiber: 5g
- Sugar: 8g

FORTIFIED PLANT-BASED SMOOTHIE

Meal Description: Fuel your day with a nutrient-packed Fortified Plant-Based Smoothie that combines the goodness of fruits, vegetables, and fortified ingredients. This smoothie is rich in vitamins, minerals, and antioxidants, making it a delicious and wholesome choice for a quick breakfast or a refreshing snack.

Ingredients:

• 1 cup fortified plant-based milk (such as almond milk or soy milk)

• 1/2 cup frozen berries (strawberries, blueberries, raspberries)

• 1/2 banana, frozen

• 1/2 cup fresh spinach leaves

• One tablespoon of almond butter or peanut butter

• One tablespoon of chia seeds or ground flaxseeds

• One scoop fortified plant-based protein powder

• Ice cubes (optional)

• Honey or maple syrup for sweetness (optional)

Instructions:

• Prepare Ingredients:

• If not using pre-frozen fruits, ensure the banana is frozen for a creamy texture. Gather all other ingredients.

• Assemble in Blender:

• Combine fortified plant-based milk, frozen berries, frozen bananas, fresh spinach leaves, almond butter or peanut butter, chia seeds, ground flaxseeds, and fortified plant-based protein powder in a blender.

• Blend Until Smooth:

• Blend the ingredients on high speed until the smoothie reaches a creamy and well-blended consistency.

• Adjust Consistency:

• If the smoothie is too thick, add more plant-based milk. If it's too thin, add additional frozen fruits or ice cubes.

• Sweeten to Taste:

• Taste the smoothie and add honey or maple syrup if additional sweetness is desired. Blend briefly to incorporate.

• Pour and Serve:

• Pour the Fortified Plant-Based Smoothie into a glass. Optionally, garnish with a sprinkle of chia seeds or a few berries.

Optional Additions:

• A handful of kale or other leafy greens for extra nutrients.

• A slice of avocado for creaminess.

• For a refreshing twist, a splash of citrus juice (orange or lemon).

Note: Customize the smoothie based on your taste

preferences and nutritional needs.

Nutrition Information (Approximate per Serving):

- Calories: 300

- Protein: 20g

- Carbohydrates: 30g

- Fat: 12g

- Saturated Fat: 1g

- Cholesterol: 0mg

- Sodium: 200mg

- Fiber: 8g

- Sugar: 15g

QUINOA AND BLACK BEAN BOWL

Meal Description: Indulge in a wholesome, protein-packed Quinoa and Black Bean Bowl for a satisfying and nutritious meal. This bowl combines the goodness of quinoa, black beans, fresh vegetables, and a zesty dressing for a flavorful and filling dish that's perfect for lunch or dinner.

Ingredients:

For the Quinoa and Black Bean Bowl:

• 1 cup quinoa, rinsed

• 2 cups water or vegetable broth

• One can (15 ounces) black beans, drained and rinsed

• 1 cup cherry tomatoes, halved

• 1 cucumber, diced

• One red bell pepper, diced

• One avocado, sliced

• Fresh cilantro, chopped, for garnish

• Lime wedges for serving

For the Zesty Dressing:

• Three tablespoons olive oil

- Two tablespoons of lime juice

- One clove of garlic, minced

- One teaspoon of ground cumin

- Salt and black pepper to taste

Instructions:

- Cook Quinoa:

- In a saucepan, combine quinoa and water or vegetable broth. Bring to a boil, then reduce heat to low, cover, and simmer for 15-20 minutes or until quinoa is cooked and water is absorbed. Fluff with a fork.

- Prepare Zesty Dressing:

- Whisk together olive oil, lime juice, minced garlic, ground cumin, salt, and black pepper in a small bowl. Set aside.

- Assemble Bowl:

- Arrange cooked quinoa, black beans, halved cherry tomatoes, diced cucumber, red bell pepper, and sliced avocado in serving bowls.

- Drizzle with Dressing:

- Drizzle the zesty dressing over the quinoa and black bean bowl.

- Garnish and Serve:

- Garnish with chopped fresh cilantro and serve with lime wedges on the side.

Optional Additions:

- Grilled corn kernels for added sweetness.

- Diced red onion for extra crunch.

• Jalapeño slices for a spicy kick.

Note: Customize the bowl with your favorite vegetables and toppings.

Nutrition Information (Approximate per Serving):

• Calories: 400

• Protein: 15g

• Carbohydrates: 55g

• Fat: 15g

• Saturated Fat: 2g

• Cholesterol: 0mg

• Sodium: 300mg

• Fiber: 12g

• Sugar: 3g

FORTIFIED NUTRITIONAL YEAST PASTA

Meal Description: Indulge in a delicious and nutrient-rich Fortified Nutritional Yeast Pasta that combines the savory goodness of nutritional yeast with whole wheat pasta and a medley of vegetables. This flavorful dish is satisfying and packed with essential vitamins and minerals. It's a wholesome option for a quick and nutritious dinner.

Ingredients:

- 8 ounces whole wheat pasta

- Two tablespoons of olive oil

- Three cloves garlic, minced

- 1 cup cherry tomatoes, halved

- 1 cup baby spinach

- 1/2 cup sliced black olives

- 1/4 cup nutritional yeast

- Salt and black pepper to taste

- Red pepper flakes for optional heat

- Fresh basil or parsley, chopped, for garnish

• Grated Parmesan cheese (optional)

Instructions:

• Cook Whole Wheat Pasta:

• Cook the whole wheat pasta according to package instructions. Drain and set aside.

• Sauté Garlic and Vegetables:

• In a large skillet, heat olive oil over medium heat. Add minced garlic and sauté until fragrant. Add halved cherry tomatoes, baby spinach, and sliced black olives. Cook until the vegetables are wilted and the tomatoes are slightly softened.

• Combine with Pasta:

• Add the cooked and drained whole wheat pasta to the skillet with the sautéed vegetables. Toss to combine.

• Add Nutritional Yeast:

• Sprinkle nutritional yeast over the pasta and vegetables. Toss well to coat evenly.

• Season and Spice:

• Season the dish with salt and black pepper to taste. Add red pepper flakes if you prefer a bit of heat.

• Garnish and Serve:

• Garnish the Fortified Nutritional Yeast Pasta with chopped fresh basil or parsley. Optionally, sprinkle grated Parmesan cheese on top.

• Serve Warm:

• Serve the pasta warm as a standalone dish or accompanied by a side salad.

Optional Additions:

• Sautéed mushrooms for added umami.

• Diced bell peppers for extra crunch and color.

• A squeeze of lemon juice for a burst of freshness.

Note: Customize the pasta with your favorite vegetables and spices.

Nutrition Information (Approximate per Serving):

• Calories: 400

• Protein: 15g

• Carbohydrates: 60g

• Fat: 10g

• Saturated Fat: 1.5g

• Cholesterol: 0mg

• Sodium: 300mg

• Fiber: 10g

• Sugar: 3g

CHICKPEA AND SPINACH CURRY

Meal Description: Savor the rich flavors of this Chickpea and Spinach Curry, a hearty and nutritious dish that brings together protein-packed chickpeas, vibrant spinach, and aromatic spices. This vegetarian curry is not only delicious but also quick and easy to prepare, making it a perfect option for a flavorful weeknight dinner.

Ingredients:

• Two cans (15 ounces each) of chickpeas, drained and rinsed

• One tablespoon of vegetable oil

• One large onion, finely chopped

• Three cloves garlic, minced

• One tablespoon of fresh ginger, grated

• One tablespoon of curry powder

• One teaspoon of ground cumin

• One teaspoon of ground coriander

• 1/2 teaspoon turmeric

• 1/2 teaspoon cayenne pepper (adjust to taste)

• One can (14 ounces) diced tomatoes

- One can (14 ounces) coconut milk

- Salt and black pepper to taste

- 4 cups fresh spinach leaves, washed

- Fresh cilantro, chopped, for garnish

- Cooked rice or naan for serving

Instructions:

- Sauté Aromatics:

- In a large skillet or pot, heat vegetable oil over medium heat. Add finely chopped onion and sauté until translucent.

- Add Garlic and Ginger:

- Stir in minced garlic and grated ginger, cooking for an additional minute until fragrant.

- Spice it Up:

- Add curry powder, cumin, coriander, turmeric, and cayenne pepper to the skillet. Stir well to coat the onions in the spices.

- Incorporate Chickpeas:

- Add drained and rinsed chickpeas to the skillet. Mix them with the spices and aromatics.

- Introduce Tomatoes and Coconut Milk:

- Pour in diced tomatoes and coconut milk. Stir to combine, and let the mixture simmer for 10-15 minutes, allowing the flavors to meld.

- Season and Add Spinach:

- Season the curry with salt and black pepper to taste. Add fresh spinach leaves to the pot and stir until wilted.

• Finish and Garnish:

• Once the spinach is wilted and the curry is heated through, taste and adjust the seasoning if needed. Garnish with fresh chopped cilantro.

• Serve:

• Serve the Chickpea and Spinach Curry over cooked rice or with naan bread.

Optional Additions:

• Squeeze of fresh lemon or lime juice for acidity.

• Diced potatoes or sweet potatoes for added texture.

• A dollop of yogurt on top for creaminess.

Note: Customize the curry to your preferred level of spiciness and thickness.

Nutrition Information (Approximate per Serving):

• Calories: 400

• Protein: 15g

• Carbohydrates: 40g

• Fat: 20g

• Saturated Fat: 15g

• Cholesterol: 0mg

• Sodium: 600mg

• Fiber: 10g

• Sugar: 5g

FORTIFIED ALMOND MILK CHIA PUDDING

Meal Description: Indulge in a nutritious and delicious Fortified Almond Milk Chia Pudding that's rich in omega-3 fatty acids, fiber, and essential vitamins. This easy-to-make chia pudding is a versatile and satisfying breakfast or snack that can be customized with your favorite toppings.

Ingredients:

• 1/4 cup chia seeds

• 1 cup fortified almond milk

• One tablespoon of maple syrup or honey (optional for sweetness)

• 1/2 teaspoon vanilla extract

• Fresh berries, sliced banana, or other fruits for topping

• Nuts, seeds, or granola for crunch (optional)

• Unsweetened coconut flakes for garnish (optional)

Instructions:

• Combine Ingredients:

• Combine chia seeds, fortified almond milk, maple syrup

or honey (if using), and vanilla extract. Stir well to ensure the chia seeds are evenly distributed.

• Refrigerate:

• Cover the bowl and refrigerate the mixture for at least 4 hours or overnight. This allows the chia seeds to absorb the liquid and create a pudding-like consistency.

• Stir Before Serving:

• Before serving, stir the chia pudding well enough to break up any clumps and achieve a smooth texture.

• Customize with Toppings:

• Spoon the chia pudding into serving bowls or jars. Top with fresh berries, sliced bananas, nuts, seeds, granola, or any toppings of your choice.

• Garnish (Optional):

• Garnish with unsweetened coconut flakes for an extra touch of flavor and texture.

• Serve and Enjoy:

• Serve the Fortified Almond Milk Chia Pudding chilled and enjoy a nutrient-packed breakfast or snack.

Optional Additions:

• A dash of cinnamon or nutmeg for warmth.

• A tablespoon of almond butter or peanut butter for added richness.

• Diced mango or pineapple for a tropical twist.

Note: Adjust the sweetness and thickness according to your taste preferences.

Nutrition Information (Approximate per Serving):

- Calories: 200
- Protein: 6g
- Carbohydrates: 20g
- Fat: 12g
- Saturated Fat: 1g
- Cholesterol: 0mg
- Sodium: 120mg
- Fiber: 10g
- Sugar: 5g

VEGAN FORTIFIED BREAKFAST BURRITO

Meal Description: Start your day with a flavorful and nutrient-packed Vegan Fortified Breakfast Burrito. This plant-based delight combines protein-rich tofu, fortified ingredients, and a medley of colorful vegetables wrapped in a tortilla for a satisfying and energizing breakfast.

Ingredients:

• One tablespoon of vegetable oil

• 1/2 block (7 ounces) firm tofu, crumbled

• 1/2 teaspoon ground turmeric

• 1/2 teaspoon smoked paprika

• Salt and black pepper to taste

• 1 cup black beans, cooked and drained

• 1 cup spinach leaves, chopped

• 1/2 cup red bell pepper, diced

• 1/4 cup red onion, finely chopped

• 1/4 cup fortified nutritional yeast

• Four whole wheat or corn tortillas

- Avocado slices for garnish

- Fresh salsa or hot sauce (optional)

Instructions:

- Sauté Tofu:

- In a skillet, heat vegetable oil over medium heat. Add crumbled tofu, ground turmeric, smoked paprika, salt, and black pepper. Sauté until the tofu is lightly browned and seasoned.

- Add Vegetables:

- Add chopped spinach, diced red bell pepper, and finely chopped red onion to the skillet. Sauté until the vegetables are tender.

- Incorporate Black Beans:

- Stir in cooked black beans and cook until everything is heated through.

- Sprinkle Nutritional Yeast:

- Sprinkle fortified nutritional yeast over the tofu and vegetable mixture. Stir to combine and let it cook for an additional minute.

- Warm Tortillas:

- Warm the tortillas in a dry skillet or microwave according to the package instructions.

- Assemble Burritos:

- Divide the tofu and vegetable mixture evenly among the tortillas. Add avocado slices on top.

- Fold and Serve:

- Fold the sides of the tortillas and roll them up to form burritos. Optionally, secure with toothpicks. Serve immediately.

• Add Salsa or Hot Sauce (Optional):

• Enhance the flavor with fresh salsa or hot sauce if desired.

Optional Additions:

• Diced tomatoes or pico de gallo for freshness.

• Jalapeño slices for extra heat.

• A squeeze of lime juice for acidity.

Note: Customize the burritos with your favorite vegan ingredients.

Nutrition Information (Approximate per Serving):

• Calories: 350

• Protein: 15g

• Carbohydrates: 40g

• Fat: 15g

• Saturated Fat: 2g

• Cholesterol: 0mg

• Sodium: 400mg

• Fiber: 10g

• Sugar: 3g

CONCLUSION

In conclusion, the role of vitamin B12 in sustaining vital bodily functions cannot be overstated. From red blood cell formation to neurological health and DNA synthesis, this essential nutrient is a linchpin for overall well-being. As we've explored, a deficiency in vitamin B12 can lead to a spectrum of health issues, ranging from anemia and neurological disorders to cognitive impairments.
Recognizing the sources of vitamin B12 is crucial, with animal products serving as the primary reservoir. While plant-based and fortified options exist, individuals following restrictive diets or facing absorption challenges must remain vigilant in ensuring adequate B12 intake. The complexity of B12 absorption, involving stomach acids and intrinsic factors, underscores the importance of a multifaceted approach to maintaining optimal levels.

Specific populations, such as vegetarians, vegans, older adults, and individuals with gastrointestinal disorders, are inherently more susceptible to B12 deficiency. For these groups, conscious dietary choices, coupled with regular monitoring and, when necessary, supplementation, become imperative in preventing the potential consequences of insufficiency.

In navigating the landscape of vitamin B12, the integration of diverse foods, fortified options, and, when needed, supplements emerges as a proactive strategy. Moreover, the collaboration between individuals and healthcare professionals remains vital for personalized guidance, early detection, and tailored interventions.

Ultimately, a well-informed approach to vitamin B12 underscores the intricate connection between diet and health. By fostering awareness, promoting diverse nutritional choices, and embracing a holistic perspective, individuals can empower themselves to address and prevent vitamin B12 deficiency, paving the way for a healthier and more resilient future.